NATURE'S PHARMACY

The Top 200 Natural Remedies

T0023091

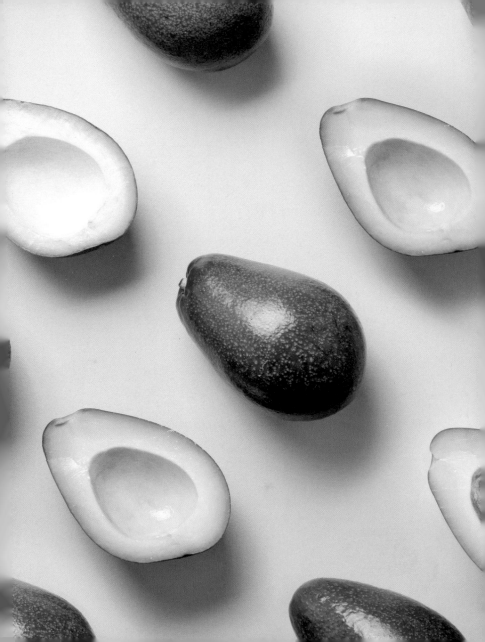

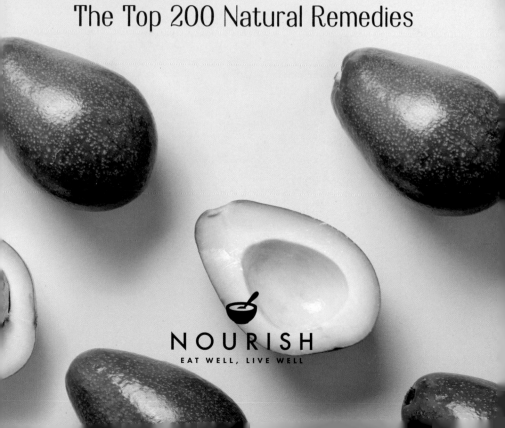

NATURE'S PHARMACY

The Top 200 Natural Remedies

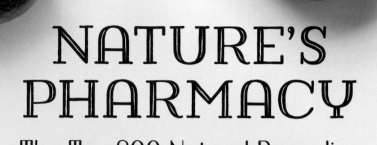

NOURISH

EAT WELL, LIVE WELL

Nature's Pharmacy
Charlotte Haigh, Anne McIntyre and Sarah Merson

First published in the USA in 2019 by
Nourish, an imprint of Watkins Media Limited.
This edition published in the UK and USA in 2021 by
Nourish, an imprint of Watkins Media Limited.
Unit 11, Shepperton House, 83–93 Shepperton Road
London N1 3DF

enquiries@nourishbooks.com

Parts of this book have previously been published in the
following volumes:
The Top 100 Immunity Boosters by Charlotte Haigh
The Top 100 Herbal Remedies by Anne McIntyre
The Top 100 Traditional Remedies by Sarah Merson

Managing Editor: Daniel Hurst
Head of Design: Glen Wilkins
Designers: Karen Smith and Kieryn Tyler
Production: Uzma Taj

A CIP record for this book is available from the British
Library

ISBN: 978-1-84899-395-2

10 9 8 7 6 5 4 3 2 1

Typeset in Helvetica Neue
Colour reproduction by XY Digital
Printed in China

Publisher's notes: While every care has been taken in
compiling the recipes for this book, Watkins Media Limited,
or any other persons who have been involved in working
on this publication, cannot accept responsibility for any
errors or omissions, inadvertent or not, that may be found
in the recipes or text, nor for any problems that may arise
as a result of preparing one of these recipes. If you are
pregnant or breastfeeding or have any special dietary
requirements or medical conditions, it is advisable to
consult a medical professional before following any of the
recipes contained in this book.

The material contained in this book is set out in good faith
for general guidance and no liability can be accepted for
loss or expense incurred in relying on the information
given. In particular this book is not intended to replace
expert medical or psychiatric advice. This book is for
informational purposes only and is for your own personal
use and guidance. It is not intended to diagnose, treat, or
act as a substitute for professional medical advice. The
author is not a medical practitioner nor a counsellor, and
professional advice should be sought if desired before
embarking on any health-related programme.

nourishbooks.com

CONTENTS

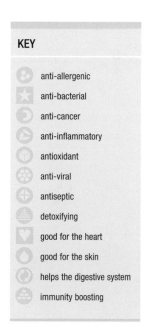

KEY

anti-allergenic

anti-bacterial

anti-cancer

anti-inflammatory

antioxidant

anti-viral

antiseptic

detoxifying

good for the heart

good for the skin

helps the digestive system

immunity boosting

Introduction

An efficient immune system is the key to maintaining good health. It helps to protect us from all manner of diseases from colds to cancer, fights food poisoning and keeps allergies in check, as well as slowing down the ageing process. But poor diet, an unhealthy lifestyle and a toxic environment can all compromise and weaken the immune system, leaving us prone to everything from common colds to more serious infections.

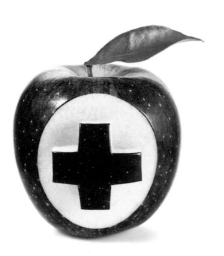

HOW THE IMMUNE SYSTEM WORKS

The immune system, which acts like a defending army, is based mainly in the lymphatic system and bloodstream, although the skin and other organs, such as the digestive system, also play an important role. The lymphatic system is a network of vessels which returns fluid from spaces between cells to the blood circulation. Lymph nodes, the spleen and the thymus gland are part of the lymph system, and they produce lymphocytes – cells which identify then set out to destroy and eliminate foreign substances, microbes and cancer cells. There are two types of lymphocytes: B-cells, and T-cells. T-cells, which are produced in the thymus, can destroy foreign bodies directly, whereas B-cells – produced in the spleen – will secrete antibodies against these undesirables in order to eliminate them. Similar to lymphocytes are natural killer cells (NK) which are particularly lethal against cancer cells, destroying them outright. The white blood cells found in the bloodstream – phagocytes and lymphocytes – play an important role in immunity by destroying invading bacteria and removing dead and damaged tissue. An optimally functioning immune system is in perfect balance. So, although it is primed to destroy foreign substances, it allows entry to those that we need, such as food. For example, the gut's immune ecology contains a balance of both friendly and unfriendly bacteria. As long as the two stay in harmony, digestive immunity is strong. But if the unfriendly bacteria start to proliferate – perhaps because your diet is high in sugar and saturated fat – you can develop digestive complaints and fungal infections.

IMMUNE-SYSTEM ENEMIES

All the immune system organs and cells rely on nutrients to keep them working efficiently. For example, interferon, an anti-viral and anti-cancer chemical secreted by tissues throughout the body, needs vitamin C for its production, while lysozyme, an anti-bacterial enzyme found in body fluids such as tears and blood, requires vitamin A. So a poor diet will result in a weakened immune system. Other enemies of strong immunity include stress, smoking, excess alcohol and caffeine, drugs (both medicinal and recreational), food additives, pesticides and pollution.

SIGNS OF LOW IMMUNITY

A poorly functioning immune system quickly makes itself known. While it's normal for most of us to have one or two colds a year, lowered immunity can make us vulnerable to every passing cold or 'flu bug, and we find ourselves succumbing to frequent infections. Other signs of inefficient immunity are digestive problems, fatigue, aching joints, muscle weakness and poor skin.

An imbalanced immune system also causes allergies and food intolerances by launching an attack when it identifies the presence of certain trigger substances. It then releases histamine and other chemicals to drive out what it perceives as an invader, causing a plethora of unwelcome symptoms.

Autoimmunity occurs when the body goes into overdrive and starts producing antibodies which attack the body's own tissues – lupus and rheumatoid arthritis are both auto-immune diseases.

Immunity-Boosting Foods

To keep the body's immune organs and cells healthy and in balance, it is vital to eat the right foods. The entire immune system needs vitamin C to function, so include plenty of foods rich in this antioxidant – most fruits and vegetables contain high levels of it. Vitamin A is powerfully anti-viral, and helps to maintain the thymus gland. It is found in liver, dairy foods, oily fish, cod liver oil and in plant foods in the form of beta-carotene, which the body then converts into vitamin A. The B-vitamins are important for

---

IMMUNITY BOOSTERS AT A GLANCE

- Foods rich in vitamins A, B complex, C and E
- Foods high in minerals, including zinc, selenium and calcium
- Omega-3 and -6 fatty acids, found in nuts, seeds and oily fish
- Protein, found in lean meat, fish and pulses
- Fibre, found in grains, pulses, fruit and vegetables
- Spending time with friends
- A positive outlook on life
- Regular exercise
- Adequate sleep
- Daylight
- Yoga and meditation

---

phagocyte (white blood cell) activity and vitamin E is a powerful antioxidant which helps stimulate antibody production.

Certain minerals are also important. Calcium helps the phagocytic cells to carry out their cleaning-up duty, while selenium is necessary for the production of antibodies. Iron builds up overall resistance, while many immune processes, including the maturation of T-cells, are heavily dependent on zinc. Most minerals can be found in seeds, nuts and green leafy vegetables.

Protein is vital for strong immunity, as it is required to manufacture all cells, including the immune system's antibodies and enzymes. It is made up of amino acids, which play a key role in immune health – for example, the amino acid glutathione is an important antioxidant and detoxifier. Many people are deficient in protein. It is important to eat plenty of protein-rich foods such as beans, pulses, meat and fish.

Other key nutrients include fibre, which is found in whole grains, fruit and vegetables. Fibre is vital for a healthy digestive system – it keeps the colon clear and prevents the build-up of toxins, and helps to prevent overgrowth of "bad" bacteria. Healthy poly-unsaturated fats are also important because they are high in omega-3 and -6 fatty acids, which reduce inflammation and boost overall immunity, so eat plenty of nuts, seeds and oily fish.

In addition to the well-known nutrients, some foods boast particular immunity enhancing properties. Green leafy vegetables, including broccoli and cabbage, contain phytochemicals called glucosinolates, which are powerfully anti-cancerous. Watermelon, pink grapefruit and tomatoes are rich in lycopene, another cancer-fighting champion, while berries such as strawberries and raspberries contain anti-inflammatory anthocyanins as well as ellagic acid, which can help to suppress the formation of cancer cells.

OTHER STEPS TO BOOST YOUR IMMUNITY

There are a number of other things that you can do, apart from eating a healthy diet, to boost your immunity. For example, you can take more exercise, which encourages the flow of lymph fluid containing immune cells around the body.

IMMUNITY ENEMIES AT A GLANCE

- A lack of vitamins and minerals
- Sugar
- Stress
- Smoking
- Excessive intake of alcohol
- Lack of exercise
- Lack of sleep

Exercise also stimulates the circulation, improving the oxygen supply to the body's organs. You don't have to go to a gym – simply staying generally active and walking briskly for half an hour every day will help. In fact, athletes are prone to poor health as rigorous over-exercising can actually suppress the immune system. The importance of having a positive attitude to life and a good social network cannot be overestimated – numerous studies have revealed that laughing, being optimistic and sharing a joke with friends can boost the immune system. Getting plenty of sleep is also important, and exposure to natural daylight is key to stimulating both mood and immunity. Yoga and meditation can release stress and help you to relax.

Traditional Remedies

"Health is the expression of a harmonious balance between various components of man's nature, the environment and ways of life ... nature is the physician of disease."

HIPPOCRATES

Traditional home remedies offer safe health treatments that have been passed down through the generations. Moreover, they can be prepared at home using plants, foods and other readily available ingredients.

In a quest to bring natural ingredients and health back into our lives, we are incorporating traditional home remedies with ever more vigour. Not only can such remedies offer tried and tested solutions to many symptoms, but they may also help us to prevent the development of ill-health in the first place.

Dating back to before ancient Egyptian times, remedies steeped in mythological and spiritual beliefs were once used as part of everyday life. They have naturally evolved over time, and have had an eventful history. The great physicians of ancient Greece – Hippocrates, Galen, Theophrastus and Dioscorides – drew on the Egyptian culture when writing their own works. Their texts were kept alive through the Dark Ages in Europe, copied by successive generations of Christian monks, and given a new lease of life with the discovery of printing in the mid-15th century. European scholars then documented and illustrated a wide variety of foods and plants, along with accounts of their remedial and hallucinatory properties, soporific and stimulating effects, and other qualities. In the 16th century European physicians such as John Gerard and Nicholas Culpeper took on a new line of work, based on the empirical observations of plants. In some cases herbal remedies began to be used in conjunction with general medicine. However, in the 1800s conventional medicine began seeking to establish a monopoly, and in a number of Western countries legislation was imposed. This banned the practice of medicine by anyone who had not been trained in a conventional medical school. Scepticism gradually set in and the medical establishment began concentrating entirely on laboratory-produced pharmaceuticals. Meanwhile, ancient remedies were deemed to be the work of mythical folklore and even witches. However, despite this resistance to them, natural remedies continued to prove their efficacy and this led to the formation of the National Institute of Medical Herbalists in 1864 – the first professional body of herbal practitioners in the world. Due to organizations such as this, traditional remedies have been afforded much of the learned wisdom of the past, as well as the benefits of modern discoveries.

For example, the ancient idea that everyday food has distinct pharmacological properties that can be used to promote health may at first seem like folklore that is decidedly deficient in the rigorous scientific proof required in the 21st century. But today, authoritative research into natural healing is progressing at a rapid pace, and traditional plant lore has proven itself with evidence of its medicinal properties. This evolution has even been encouraged by the scientific community, which is increasingly recognizing the numerous benefits of plants and other natural substances through experimentation and experience.

ANCIENT MEDICINAL REMEDIES

• The ancient Egyptians were the first to use a method known as "infusion" to extract the oils from aromatic plants.

• The early Aztecs used garlic to prevent tuberculosis.

• The Romans cured hiccups by consuming small amounts of raw cabbage in vinegar.

• The Romans took much of their medical knowledge from the Greeks, and then refined the use of many remedies.

• During the building of the pyramids, Egyptian workers were given garlic daily to rid them of spirits and give them the vitality and strength to perform well.

• It was a Roman tradition to use the yolks of eggs, mixed with the ash of their shells, for dysentery.

• The Aztecs once smeared avocado pulp on sexual organs to enhance sexual appetite.

• The Egyptians mixed together the fats of lion, hippo, cat, crocodile and serpent to anoint the head of a bald person and stimulate hair growth.

THE USE OF NATURAL THERAPEUTICS IN A CHANGING WORLD

There exists a real alchemy with the majority of ingredients used in traditional remedies. For example, plants take from the soil essential nutritive substances that they then store and convert into usable forms. They are, therefore, natural reservoirs of precious elements drawn from the soil, which past generations have had the wisdom and down-to-earth common sense to make good use of. Unfortunately, since the Industrial Revolution many of the soils in developed countries have changed dramatically. This, in turn, has led to a decline in the quality of our food. In order to get the best from nature's garden, we need to be reminded of the practices our ancestors observed:

• Look to Mother Nature – remember plants growing in the wild are a product of nature and therefore have more innately potent properties than those of modern cultivated varieties.

• When selecting plants it is preferable to choose from those that are growing some distance apart, rather than those tightly packed together.

• Always choose fruits, vegetables and herbs that have the most fragrance, taste and colour. These are the ones that are also the most fresh and nutritive.

NATUROPATHIC GUIDELINES FOR BETTER HEALTH

• Lead a wholesome lifestyle.
• Eat organic, unadulterated food.
• Eat local, seasonal produce whenever possible.
• Eat slowly, chewing food thoroughly.
• Avoid processed and junk food.
• Drink 2 litres (70fl oz/8½ cups) of pure, clean water each day.
• Try to detox your body twice a year.

• Wear clothing made from natural fibres and dyes.
• Choose skin-care products free of chemicals, foaming agents, etc.
• Always use natural deodorants rather than chemical anti-perspirants.
• Make sure you get plenty of sunlight.
• Stimulate circulation and excretion of toxins through daily skin brushing.

• Get plenty of rest and relaxation to maintain your body's inherent healing mechanisms.
• Exercise for at least 30 minutes 3–4 times a week – walking, yoga, Pilates and tai chi are all examples of good types of exercise.
• Try to achieve a healthy life balance: take time out to relax in the company of your family and friends.

TOWARDS SELF-HEALING

It may no longer be necessary for us to go foraging in the woods and hedgerows, or to hunt wild animals as our ancestors did. Today, many ingredients that were hunted and gathered by our forefathers are commonly available in health-food stores and even supermarkets, and they can do much to help us live healthy lives.

We know that many natural ingredients have proven medicinal value, as well as providing sustenance, yet the dividing line between "food" and "medicine" is not always clear. However, we have learned that when it comes to healing, they are, in fact, part of the same thing. Moreover, such is the way of traditional remedies that – whether they are ingested internally or used topically – the body will take what it needs from the food or plant with the ultimate goal of rebalancing the system. This union with nature ultimately allows us to regain our own innate ability to heal ourselves.

While our lifestyles are very different from those of our ancestors, traditional remedies – which are innately nurturing and healing – can have huge benefits on our current hurried lifestyles, and we need them more today than we have ever done.

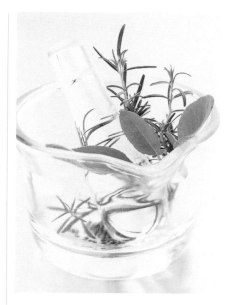

This book provides details of some of the most important properties of 100 of the best natural ingredients that can be used to maintain and often improve health. Symbols supplementing the text give at-a-glance information on the key properties of each ingredient described.

The use of traditional remedies places every aspect of health back in our own hands and leaves little doubt that it is worth rediscovering our roots.

Herbs – The Original Medicine

Herbs have always been central to our lives. The plant world provides us with the foods we enjoy and the air we breathe. It is hardly surprising therefore that it supplies us with remedies for treating our everyday ills, too; cultures all over the world have used these remedies for thousands of years. Our kitchen cupboards, our gardens and our hedgerows are full of potent medicines for almost every common ailment.

We have much to thank our ancestors for. Their insights into the successful use of indigenous foods and plants as medicines have survived through generations to give us a rich, global heritage of herbal medicine. The earliest records of herbal medicine originate from China and date back to around 2500BCE. The Ebers Papyrus from Egypt, which dates from around 1500BCE, mentions more than 700 herbal remedies, many of which are still popular today. We know that several other peoples – notably the Greeks, Persians, Indians and Aztecs – used medicinal plants beyond 1000BCE. These plants have provided the source for our medicines ever since.

However, in the second half of the nineteenth century, the rapid development of science and chemistry saw a steep decline in the popularity of herbs. Chemists began to isolate and extract the therapeutically active substances within the herbs and soon the tradition of healing using the whole plant fell away. Before long, scientists were able to manufacture synthetic versions of these active ingredients and the herbs, which had been revered for so long, were viewed as old-fashioned and obsolete.

Nevertheless, despite the use of sophisticated drugs and our modern-day calls for scientific proof in everything, in the last 20 years we have witnessed an enormous surge in interest in herbal medicine. Indeed, traditional plant remedies continue to provide around 85 per cent

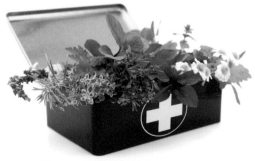

of the world's medicines. They are just as valuable today as they ever were.

MODERN MEDICINE'S DEBT TO HERBS

From a "scientific" point of view, many herbal medicines are considered to be experimental and unreliable. However, humanity has been using herbal medicines safely and successfully for thousands of years. Scientists developed many of the familiar and potent medicines of the twenty-first century from herbs, the constituents of which have provided the blueprint for many of the most effective and widely known drugs in use today. For example, quinine, the anti-malaria drug, is extracted from cinchona, found in the bark of a South-American tree; vincristine, the anti-tumour drug, comes from the Madagascan periwinkle; morphine and codeine come from the beautiful opium poppy. Atropine, aspirin, digoxin and ephedrine are all plant-derived drugs of unquestionable value. Long before the discovery of modern antibiotics, echinacea – a beautiful plant of the daisy family – was one of the most commonly prescribed remedies for infections. Of course, we now know for sure that echinacea can boost the activity of our immune system.

Since the nineteenth century, the chemical analysis of plants has laid the foundations of a more scientific approach to herbalism. As interest into herbal medicine increases, scientists are undertaking a corresponding amount of research. All over the world they are looking into the properties of more and more foods and herbs in the belief that they will provide new cures for illnesses such as heart disease and cancer. They are making exciting discoveries that support our ancient ancestors' beliefs in herbal treatments: remedies such as ginger for arthritis and turmeric for gout, have been found to have scientific merit after all; to have a basis in fact, not merely in folklore.

In the first few years of their renewed popularity, herbs were hailed as miracle remedies and panaceas, and because they are "natural" they were said to be devoid of the side-effects of orthodox medicines. A rebound effect then followed: far from championing herbal remedies, one article after another began to raise concerns about their safety. With insufficient real evidence to guide them, the public and professionals alike are susceptible to media hype. However, my great hope is that as more up-to-date, accurate information becomes readily available, we will all learn that herbal remedies are immensely effective – but only if we use them correctly. Anyone using herbs needs to be aware of their possible risks as well as their benefits.

Nevertheless the empirical evidence gathered over thousands of years, and proven by recent research, means that those who want to use herbs may rest assured that the medicine of the herbalist is based on strong foundations. Today's herbalists have the best of both worlds: their practice is based on a thorough knowledge of the traditional uses of plant medicines, as well as constantly updated scientific research.

USING THE WHOLE PLANT

Until recently the world of science has regarded plants merely as a source of active ingredients, made up of chemicals that can be separated out, analyzed and assessed in terms of biochemistry. As scientists put plants under the microscope and identified their active ingredients, they isolated single constituents, which they then used to replace whole-plant medicines. The belief of pharmacologists was that if a man-made product was similar to one derived from the plant world, the body would assimilate it in a similar way. In addition they believed that the man-made version was, in fact, superior to the natural constituent of a plant, because it was not subject to the relatively random laws of nature. Essentially, because its active ingredients were more easily measured, the man-made dosage was more reliable. Herbalists, on the other hand, prefer to treat their patients using the whole plant, believing this to be a gentler and safer form of treatment. They believe that, by isolating and synthesizing potent active ingredients, man-made remedies are likely to increase the risk of toxicity in the body and create unwanted side-effects. Another herbalist's maxim is "the whole plant is greater than the sum of its constituent parts".

There are two different types of substance found in medicinal plants, and each has an important role to play in the healing process. The primary healing agents are the active ingredients that the early chemists were interested in extracting. Most healing plants contain several active substances, one of which will be dominant. It is this dominant ingredient that influences the choice of plant by the herbal practitioner when making up a prescription for a patient. The secondary healing agents are substances such as hormones, enzymes and trace elements. We should never underestimate the importance of the secondary healing agents, because without them the active substances could have totally different effects on the body. Secondary agents act as catalysts, enhancing the action of the plants by ensuring that the body adequately absorbs and assimilates all the active constituents – dominant or otherwise. At the same time the secondary agents buffer the active constituents' more powerful actions in a variety of ways to prevent side-effects. It is the natural combination of both types of substance that determines the healing power and safety of the herbal medicines we use.

There is no better way to illustrate this than by examples – and the world of herbs is full of them. Take meadowsweet: this plant, with pretty white flowers, contains salicylic acid, which is the plant's active constituent and has an action that is similar to aspirin. It is widely known that aspirin itself can cause internal bleeding in people with sensitive stomach linings. However, herbalists actually use meadowsweet to treat an inflamed or bleeding stomach lining. The plant's secondary agents include tannin and mucilage, both of which act to protect and heal the mucous membrane of the stomach. So, while aspirin's side-effects go unchecked; meadowsweet has its own internal balancer. To illustrate this point further, most diuretic drugs (which promote urination) cause the body to lose potassium. As a result when doctors prescribe diuretics, they also need to prescribe a potassium supplement to rectify the imbalance. Herbalists use dandelion leaves as a diuretic. These leaves are themselves rich in potassium, thus combining a non-toxic diuretic with an integral potassium supplement. Finally, ephedra (*Ephedra sinica*) is a plant that the Chinese have used for thousands of years for its medicinal benefits. In relatively modern times chemists have extracted the alkaloid ephedrine from the plant, which doctors today prescribe as a treatment for myriad conditions, including nasal congestion, bronchial coughs, and asthma. Some reports claim that on its own ephedrine raises blood pressure. In the whole ephedra plant there are six other alkaloids, and the predominant one actually prevents any increase in blood pressure or in heart rate. Time and again we can see that the isolated active constituents can have serious side-effects on our well-being; while the whole plant keeps itself, and us, in balance.

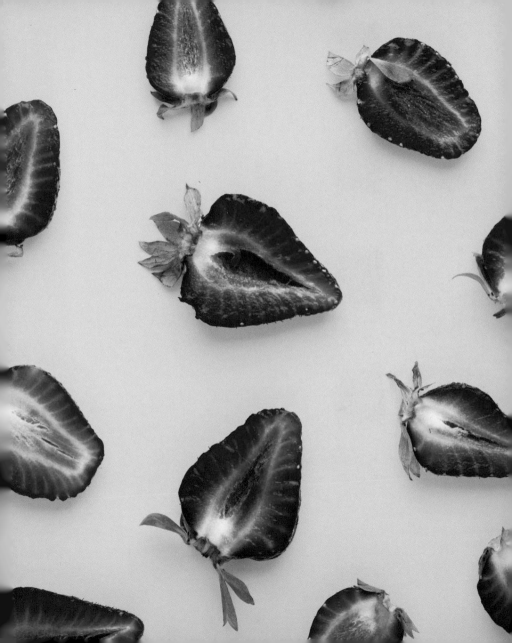

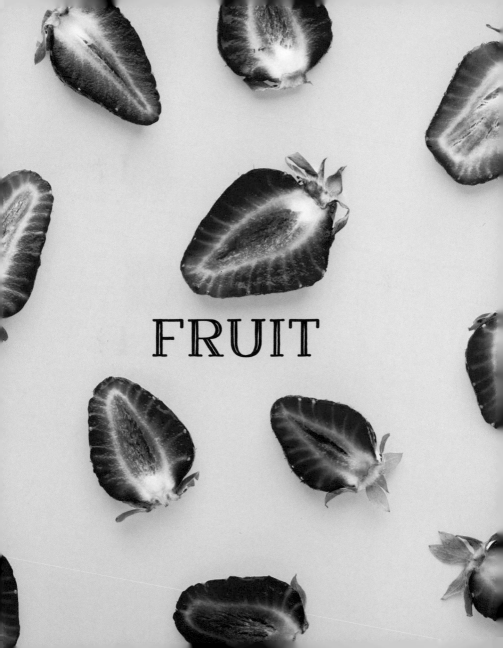

FRUIT

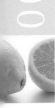

Lemon

PROPERTIES/ACTIONS
- Strengthening
- Extracting
- Boosts immunity
- Liver stimulant

PARTS USED
- Whole fruit

LEMON POULTICE
for boils & abscesses

1 lemon, sliced
gauze bandage

Use the bandage to tie a slice
of lemon against the boil or
abscess. A hot-water bottle
can be used to apply heat,
if desired. Leave for about
10 minutes, then discard.
Repeat 2 or 3 times a day until
the boil opens and drains.

**Used originally by the Romans to sweeten the
breath, lemons are packed full of nutrients and
are used today to treat a number of ailments.**

Lemons are rich in citrus flavonoids such as vitamin C, and have
important antioxidant functions. They can strengthen the immune
system, assist the healing of wounds and strengthen the walls of
blood capillaries. Because of their antiseptic qualities, lemons are
used to treat infections of the respiratory tract. Their dissolving and
extracting qualities help in the topical treatment of boils and
abscesses. Lemons are also a liver stimulant, and can therefore be
used for detoxification – for example, when drank as lemon water.

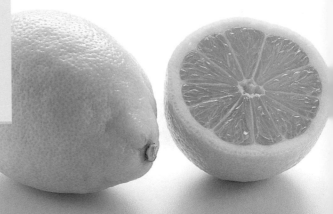

Orange

This popular and versatile citrus fruit is bursting with immunity-boosting vitamins.

Oranges are one of the top sources of vitamin C, which is crucial for strong immunity, helping to fight viruses, produce disease-fighting cells, and battle bacteria. They also contain beta-sitosterol, a plant sterol that has been shown to help prevent tumour formation and to lower blood cholesterol. In addition, oranges also contain vitamin B5, which helps to stimulate immune response, and are high in the fibre needed for a healthy heart and digestive system.

NUTRIENTS
Vitamins B3, B5, C, carotenoids, folate; beta-sitosterol, potassium; fibre

TANGY PANCAKES *serves 4*

1 egg
150ml (5fl oz/⅔ cup) skimmed milk
70g (2½oz/½ cup) plain (all-purpose) flour
2 oranges
1 tbsp raw cane sugar
a knob of unsalted butter
4 tbsp plain bio-yogurt

Beat together the egg and milk, then fold in the flour and grated zest of one orange. Peel both the oranges, and divide them into segments. Put these in a saucepan. Add the sugar, and cook over a low heat for 2 minutes. Melt a little butter in a frying pan, then add a quarter of the batter mixture for each pancake, cooking until golden brown, turning once. Serve with the oranges and the yogurt.

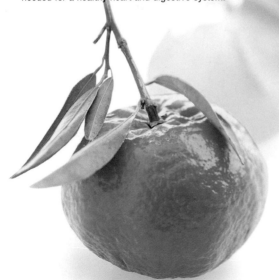

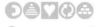

Grapefruit

NUTRIENTS

Vitamin C, beta-carotene, folic acid
(folate); potassium; lycopene;
flavonoids; fibre

**This sharp and tangy breakfast fruit is detoxifying
and immune-strengthening.**

The grapefruit is thought to have originated in the West Indies
before reaching the rest of the world in the 18th century. There
are several different varieties, including sour-tasting
yellow ones, and the sweeter pink and ruby-red types.

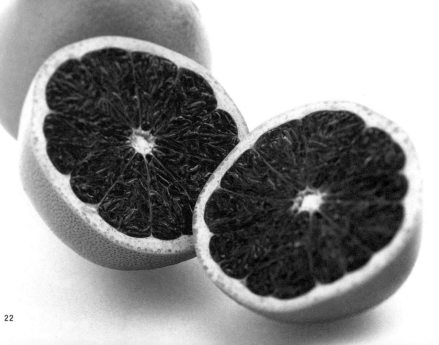

GRAPEFRUIT'S IMMUNITY-BOOSTING PROPERTIES

Every part of a grapefruit is a powerful detoxifier. Its high vitamin C content enhances immunity and tissue growth, and the flesh and rind are thought to contain compounds that help to inhibit cancer development. The pulp is high in pectin, a soluble fibre that binds with excess cholesterol to remove it from the body, and helps to eliminate toxins and waste, relieving constipation. Its seeds contain an anti-parasite, anti-fungal compound which, although not edible whole, can be taken in supplement form (grapefruit seed extract).

USING GRAPEFRUIT

The sweet pink variety, which is richer in beta-carotene, is the best option for those who dislike bitter flavours. Grapefruit is delicious eaten on its own, cut in half so that the flesh can be scooped out. It also works well juiced, either alone or in combination with other fruit, such as apple or raspberries, although juicing removes the fibre content.

GRAPEFRUIT FACTS

• Grapefruit juice can enhance the action of certain prescribed drugs, including some sleeping pills, so check with your doctor if you are taking medication.

• The white pith that lines the skin and divides the segments is thought to be particularly rich in pectin, so eat this to gain the full benefits for your heart.

• The scent of grapefruit has been found to suppress the appetite and lift the mood – try adding a couple of drops of grapefruit essential oil to a tissue and sniffing it.

STUFFED GRAPEFRUIT *serves 4*

2 grapefruits, halved, flesh removed and chopped
1 avocado, peeled, pitted and cubed
2.5cm (1in) piece fresh ginger, chopped
1 pear, peeled, cored and cubed

1 green (bell) pepper, deseeded and chopped
2 black olives, pitted and halved
2 tbsp lemon balm, finely chopped

Mix the grapefruit flesh with the avocado, ginger, pear and green pepper, and divide the filling among the 4 halves. Garnish with the olives and lemon balm, and serve.

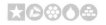

Apricot

As their bright orange colour shows, apricots are rich in beta-carotene. They have been prominent in Indian and Chinese folklore for 2,000 years.

PROPERTIES/ACTIONS
- Balancing
- Supports respiratory tract
- Rich in iron

PARTS USED
- Whole fruit

APRICOT MASSAGE OIL
for dry, sensitive skins

**250g (9oz) apricot seeds
750ml (26fl oz/3 cups)
carrier oil**

With a pestle and mortar, grind the seeds to release the oils, then place them in a clear glass jar. Pour the carrier oil onto the seeds, secure and shake. Place in a sunny spot and leave for 2 to 6 weeks. Pour the oil through a sieve lined with muslin (cheesecloth) into a jug, then pour into dark glass bottles. Store for up to a year. Apply liberally to the skin when needed.

Apricots have high levels of beta-carotene, which the body turns into anti-viral vitamin A. Eating fresh apricots can be helpful to those suffering from infection, particularly infections of the respiratory tract. Dried apricots supply iron and produce haemoglobin, which is beneficial to those suffering from anaemia. They also have a balancing effect on the nervous system, treating mental fatigue, mild anxiety and insomnia, and yield an oil that is highly nourishing and protective to the skin.

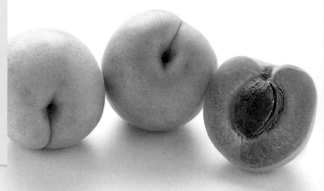

Apple

Over the course of centuries, apple has acquired a reputation as a healthful fruit and remedy, thus confirming the old adage, "An apple a day keeps the doctor away."

Stimulating the liver and kidneys, apples have a detoxifying effect on the body. They are rich in pectin, which binds to and helps dispel toxins and cholesterol, and malic acid, which neutralizes acid by-products. Apples may treat constipation and diarrhoea. They slow the rise of blood sugar and help control diabetes. Containing quercetin, an anti-inflammatory, apples lower the risk of heart disease and are useful in the treatment of arthritis and allergic reactions.

PROPERTIES/ACTIONS
- Dispels toxins
- Controls blood sugar
- Anti-inflammatory

PARTS USED
- Whole fruit

In Greek mythology, golden versions of apple grew on trees guarded by the Hesperides.

AGE-OLD APPLE & LIQUORICE INFUSION
for gastric, kidney & pulmonary conditions

2–3kg (4½–6½lb) apples, unpeeled and thinly sliced into rounds
2 small pieces liquorice root

Place the apples in a saucepan and cover with 1 litre (35fl oz/ 4 cups) water. Add the liquorice root and boil for 15 minutes, then strain and discard the apple and liquorice. Drink throughout the day.

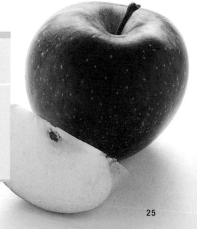

Plum

This versatile fruit can be eaten fresh or dried, and is a useful source of immunity-boosting antioxidants.

NUTRIENTS

Vitamins B2, C, beta-carotene; copper, potassium

Plums are rich in pectin, a type of soluble fibre that absorbs and neutralizes toxins in the large intestine, which means that they have excellent detoxifying properties. They're great for helping to improve fitness in anaemia-prone athletes because they're packed with iron, which is crucial in the formation of red blood cells. They also contain malic acid and the antioxidant vitamin C, both of which enhance the absorption of iron.

PLUM COMPÔTE

16 ripe but firm plums
2 tsp ground allspice
2 tbsp dark brown sugar
250ml (9fl oz/1 cup) orange juice
zest of ½ orange
plain bio-yogurt, to serve

Place the plums in a large ovenproof dish. Add the allspice, sugar, orange juice and zest, and bake in a pre-heated oven at 180°C/350°F/Gas 4 for 30 minutes. Serve with bio-yogurt.

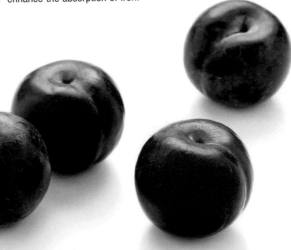

Peach

This deliciously sweet treat helps to prevent dehydration – a common cause of fatigue.

A 2-per-cent loss of fluid can cause a 20-per-cent drop in energy, which is why dehydration is one of the major causes of fatigue during prolonged exercise. As well as drinking plenty of water, eating foods with a high water content, such as a ripe, juicy peach, is a good way to top up fluids. Peaches also contain the trace mineral boron, which affects the way the body metabolizes calcium and so is important for healthy bones.

Avoid buying peaches that have a green tinge, as they will never ripen properly.

NUTRIENTS
Vitamins B3, C, beta-carotene, folic acid (folate); calcium, iron, magnesium, phosphorus, potassium, zinc

PEACHY FROZEN YOGURT

4 peaches, peeled and pitted
10 raspberries
10 strawberries, hulled
300ml (10½fl oz/1¼ cups)
   natural bio-yogurt
juice of ½ lemon

Purée the fruit in a blender and place in a bowl in the freezer for 2–3 hours until semi-frozen. Remove and whisk in the yogurt and lemon juice. Freeze again until firm. Remove from the freezer 30 minutes before serving.

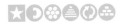

Guava

NUTRIENTS

Vitamins B3, C, beta-carotene; fibre

This highly-scented tropical treat is exceptionally high in vitamin C, and an effective detoxifier.

Guava gets its deep orange colour from beta-carotene, which the body turns into vitamin A. Important for keeping viruses at bay and helping to prevent cancer, vitamin A is a powerful antioxidant that works with vitamin C to mop up damaging free radicals and keep the body's organs healthy. Guava is rich in fibre and has detoxifying properties. In addition it can help to calm autoimmune disorders, such as rheumatoid arthritis.

Guava acts as an immune system stimulant, helping to trigger immune response.

GUAVA CRUSH

1 guava, peeled and diced
1 small orange, peeled and
    segmented
2 green apples, diced
1 slice of lime, to decorate

Press the ingredients through a juicer. Serve with ice and garnished with a slice of lime.

Papaya

First used in Mayan medicine, papayas have beautiful yellow-orange flesh and are packed with carotenoids, helpful for many diseases.

Papaya comes out on top in the antioxidant stakes, with half a fruit providing a whopping 38 milligrams of powerful carotenoids. It can thus help to protect against cancer and cardiovascular disease, and to treat skin irritations.

Papaya contains protease enzymes similar to those present in the stomach, therefore favouring healthy digestion. The fruit is a mild diuretic, and is particularly useful in treating children's urinary and digestive ailments.

PROPERTIES/ACTIONS
- Protective
- Promotes healthy digestion
- Diuretic

PARTS USED
- Whole fruit

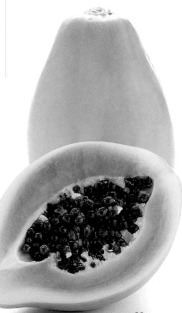

PAPAYA-MINT SALSA

1 under-ripe papaya, peeled and
   deseeded
3 small carrots, peeled
4 spring onions (scallions)
1 lemon and 2 limes
4 drops green Tabasco sauce
2 tsp vegetable oil
1 tsp salt
pinch of black pepper
15g (½oz/⅓ cup) coarsely
   chopped mint leaves

Finely chop the papaya, carrots and spring onions and place in a bowl. Toss together. Using a sharp knife, remove the peel and pith from the lemon. Section and chop the lemon and 1 lime. Add to the mixture, then squeeze the juice from the remaining lime into the bowl. Add the Tabasco sauce, oil, salt, pepper and mint. Toss together to combine.

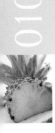

Pineapple

PROPERTIES/ACTIONS
- Reduces inflammation
- Speeds tissue repair
- Protects bones
- Energizing

PARTS USED
- Whole fruit

Inside their tough skins, fresh pineapples have "hearts of gold": they are rich in bromelain, vitamin C and manganese.

Containing the enzyme bromelain, pineapple has a centuries-old reputation for its anti-inflammatory action. It is useful in treating conditions from sinusitis and rheumatoid arthritis, to sore throats and gout. It may help speed recovery from injuries and surgery, help alleviate fluid retention, and prevent blood clots and conditions such as arteriosclerosis. Bromelain can help the gut to operate efficiently and effectively, and is therefore a useful remedy for digestive problems. The vitamin C content in pineapples helps to thwart free radicals and boost immunity. Vitamin C also helps to

PINEAPPLE PEEL REMEDY *for dry, dead skin*

1 small pineapple
first-aid tape or light bandage

Soak the dry skin area in a bowl of warm water for 20 minutes. Cut a piece of pineapple peel and place it flesh side-down directly on the skin. Secure the peel with tape and leave overnight. Carefully remove the dressing, then soak the skin in water for 5 minutes. Repeat for approximately 4 consecutive nights.

PINEAPPLE & HONEY MARINADE *for salmon or chicken*

200g (7oz) pineapple, peeled and finely chopped
2 garlic cloves, crushed
1–2 tbsp honey
1 tsp ground allspice
1 tsp freshly ground nutmeg
1 tsp ground cinnamon
1 tsp ground cloves
pinch of salt

Mix together all the ingredients and leave to stand for 15 minutes. Pour over the salmon or chicken and leave to marinade for 2 hours, before cooking.

make bone-protecting collagen, and pineapples are a good source of manganese, which also makes collagen. Used topically, the bromelain content of pineapple can help to soften dead skin.

In ancient Indian medicine pineapples were thought to act as a uterine tonic.

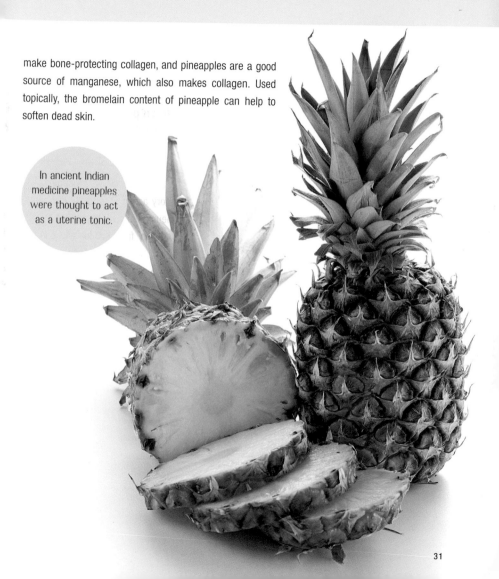

011

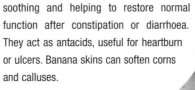

Banana

PROPERTIES/ACTIONS
- Nourishing
- Energizing
- Soothing

PARTS USED
- Whole fruit

BANANA SKIN POULTICE
for corns & calluses

2 small, unripe banana skins strip of cloth

Using the cloth, bandage a piece of unripe banana skin, gummy-side down, onto the corn. Leave overnight and discard in the morning. Repeat the following night. After 2 days soak the feet in hot water, then scrape away the softened corn with a pumice stone. Repeat as necessary.

Bananas are packed with nourishing nutrients, particularly the mineral potassium, and have a long history of use as a natural energizer.

Because bananas are rich in potassium, they are a great energy food. They lower blood pressure and protect against heart disease by maintaining fluid balance and preventing plaque from sticking to artery walls. Bananas are also rich in fibre, and are therefore highly beneficial to the digestive tract, soothing and helping to restore normal function after constipation or diarrhoea. They act as antacids, useful for heartburn or ulcers. Banana skins can soften corns and calluses.

The horticulture employed on banana plantations has its origins in prehistoric times.

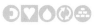

Cantaloupe Melon

NUTRIENTS
Vitamins B3, C, beta-carotene

This summer melon takes its name from the town of Cantaloupe near Rome.

Cantaloupe melon is one of the richest sources of beta-carotene, which the body converts to vitamin A, an antioxidant that is crucial for the production of disease-fighting lymphocyte cells. This fruit is also rich in vitamin C, which we need for all immune functions and to protect us against colds, cancer, and heart disease. Its high water content gives it a mildly diuretic action, helping to detoxify the body.

RED MELON SALAD
serves 4

2 Cantaloupe melons, peeled, deseeded and cubed
1 pink grapefruit, divided into segments
10 raspberries
2.5cm (1in) piece fresh ginger, grated

Combine the melon and grapefruit pieces in a large bowl and leave for 30 minutes to allow the juices to mingle. Divide into 4 serving bowls and garnish with the raspberries and the ginger.

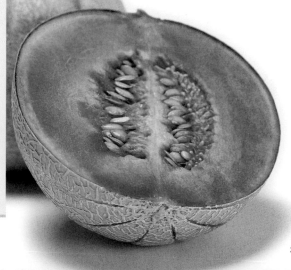

013

Pear

Bursting with natural sugar that converts easily into energy, a pear is an ideal pre-workout snack.

One pear contains approximately one-tenth of the recommended daily intake of potassium, a mineral easily lost through perspiration. This is important for anyone who exercises because a lack of potassium can lead to fatigue and muscle cramps. Pears are also among the few fruits that contain lots of insoluble fibre, which works like tiny scrubbing brushes in the colon to promote good digestion.

NUTRIENTS

Vitamin C, beta-carotene, folic acid (folate); calcium, iron, magnesium, phosphorus, potassium, zinc

POACHED PEARS

4 pears, peeled
100g (3½oz/6 tbsp) clear honey
125ml (4½fl oz/½ cup) apple juice
1 tsp ground ginger

Place the pears in a pan and pour over the honey, juice and 250ml (9fl oz/1 cup) water. Sprinkle over the ginger and bring to the boil. Reduce the heat, cover and simmer for 20 minutes. Allow to cool in the syrup.

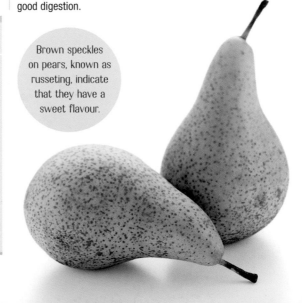

Brown speckles on pears, known as russeting, indicate that they have a sweet flavour.

Mango

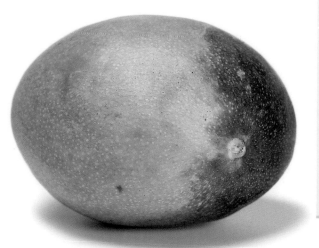

Regarded by many as the most delicious tropical fruit, mango is also crammed full of nutrients.

Mango is an excellent source of beta-carotene, the precursor to anti-viral vitamin A. It also contains high levels of vitamin C, which is crucial for good overall immune function. This increasingly popular exotic fruit is one of the few fruit sources of vitamin E, an important antioxidant which helps to fight damaging free radicals in the body, as well as boosting the action of disease-battling antibodies.

NUTRIENTS
Vitamins B3, C, E, beta-carotene; fibre

Mango is perfect in fruit salads and desserts, but it works equally well in savoury dishes.

MANGO SMOOTHIE
serves 2

**1 mango, peeled, pitted and sliced
½ pineapple, peeled, cored and chopped
10 strawberries, hulled
75ml (2½fl oz/⅓ cup) pineapple juice
75ml (2½fl oz/⅓ cup) plain bio-yogurt**

Place all the ingredients in a blender and whizz until smooth and creamy. Serve immediately.

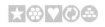

Lime

High in vitamin C, the tangy flesh of lime is an effective immune stimulant.

NUTRIENTS

Vitamin C, folic acid (folate); calcium, potassium; fibre

TANGY CITRUS JUICE

serves 1–2

2 oranges
1 grapefruit
1 lemon
1 lime

Peel and slice the fruits, and press alternate pieces of each through a juicer. Drink immediately.

Lime has high levels of immune-essential vitamin C. It has powerful anti-viral properties and triggers the production of phagocytes, which mop up the invaders that cause disease, as well as fighting bacteria. The vitamin C content keeps the immune system balanced and soothes allergic reactions. Lime is also a good source of folate, which is needed for healthy DNA formation and reproductive function, and contains fibre, which helps to keep cholesterol levels low and prevent heart disease.

Lime can help to speed up the body's natural healing process.

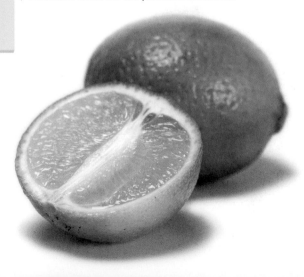

Kiwi Fruit

Containing more vitamin C than oranges, kiwi fruit is a top immunity booster.

Kiwi fruit's immunity-enhancing abilities lie mainly in its super-dose of vitamin C. Just one fruit contains around 120 per cent of an adult's daily recommended intake, and unlike many other fruits, the nutrients remain intact long after harvesting, with 90 per cent of its vitamin C content still present after 6 months' storage. Kiwi fruit is also a good source of fibre, which we need for an efficient digestive system and a healthy heart.

NUTRIENTS
Vitamins B3, C, beta-carotene; fibre

Kiwi fruit can cause allergic reactions in some children.

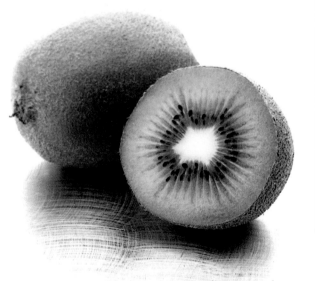

TROPICAL FRUIT SALAD
serves 4

4 kiwi fruits, peeled and sliced
1 mango, peeled, pitted and cubed
1 papaya, peeled, deseeded and sliced
8 lychees, peeled, pitted and halved
1 pineapple, peeled and cubed
pulp of 4 passion fruits

Combine all the ingredients together in a large bowl. Leave for an hour for the juices to mingle, then serve.

Raspberry

Raspberries are high in antioxidants and other protective nutrients essential for good health, and are commonly used as a home remedy.

PROPERTIES/ACTIONS
- Astringent
- Treats diarrhoea
- Uterine relaxant

PARTS USED
- Whole fruit & leaves

According to folklore raspberries have the ability to soothe inflamed tonsils.

This tart fruit contains a host of absorbable nutrients, from vitamin C to calcium, potassium, iron and magnesium, all of which are essential to the convalescent, as well as to those suffering from heart problems, fatigue and depression.

Raspberries are naturally astringent and can therefore help to treat upset stomachs and diarrhoea. An infusion made of raspberry leaves can facilitate labour by acting as both a uterine relaxant and a tonic.

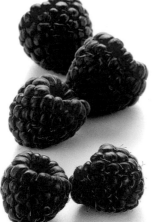

RASPBERRY LEAF TEA *for painful periods or to facilitate labour*

60g (2¼ oz/4 cups) young
  raspberry leaves, or 25g (1oz/
  2 cups) dried leaves
500ml (16fl oz/2 cups) freshly
  boiled water

Put the leaves in a large cup and pour over the boiling water. Cover and leave to stand for 15 minutes, then strain. Drink up to 5 cups a day. Caution: use only from week 32 of pregnancy.

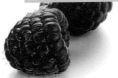

Strawberry

Strawberries enhance liver and gallbladder functions, and are a traditional remedy for treating gout, arthritis and kidney stones.

The Romans used strawberries to relieve everything from loose teeth to gastritis.

Extremely high in antioxidants, strawberries contain ellagic acid, which is believed to help cellular changes leading to cancer. They are a good source of vitamin C, and can thus help to fight infection and heart disease. Their high iron content makes them therapeutic for anaemia and fatigue. Strawberries are a mild laxative and antibacterial, and may help to regenerate intestinal flora. They can also dissolve tartarous incrustations on the teeth.

PROPERTIES/ACTIONS
- Astringent
- Diuretic
- Nervine

PARTS USED
- Whole fruit & leaves

STRAWBERRY & HONEY DECOCTION *for sore throats*

30g (1oz/⅙ cup) strawberries
30g (1oz/1 cup) strawberry leaves
honey, to taste

Place all the ingredients, except the honey, in an aluminium or stainless steel pan with 750ml (26fl oz/3 cups) water. Bring to the boil and simmer, uncovered, for about 15 minutes to reduce. Add the honey. Strain and discard the ingredients. Transfer to a glass bottle with a lid and store in the refrigerator. Gargle 150ml (5fl oz/²/₃ cup) of the mixture every 30 minutes.

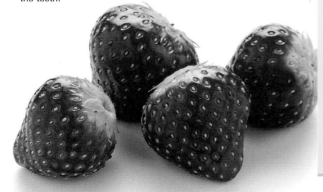

★ ➲ ◈

Cranberry

Due to their antibacterial properties, cranberries have become a renowned remedy for treating infections of the urinary tract and kidney stones.

PROPERTIES/ACTIONS
- Supports urinary tract
- Fights infection

PARTS USED
- Whole fruit

CRANBERRY-ORANGE RELISH

300g (12oz/2 cups)
   cranberries, fresh or frozen
1 medium orange, unpeeled,
   cut into eighths and deseeded
1 apple, unpeeled, cut into
   eighths and cored
75g (2½oz/⅓ cup)
   granulated sugar
1 tsp ground ginger

Blend the fruit in a food processor. Stir in the sugar and ginger, and transfer to a glass jar. Cover with a lid and refrigerate for at least 4 hours. Use when needed.

Cranberries are a valuable source of vitamin C, and the Native Americans first introduced Europeans to cranberries to help combat scurvy. It became recognized that the acidity of cranberries increases the natural acidity of urine, thus preventing bacteria from thriving. Cranberries are therefore very effective against cystitis. Being rich in antioxidants, cranberries may also help to ward off colds and other diseases, including some cancers.

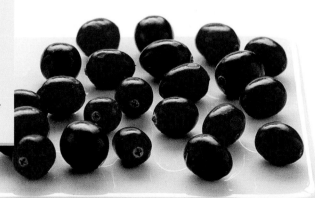

Goji Berry

NUTRIENTS
Vitamins B1, B2, B6, C, E, beta-carotene, folic acid (folate); calcium, iron, phosphorus, potassium, selenium, zinc; omega-3 and omega-6 essential fatty acids

SWEET POTATO AND GOJI BERRY FRITTERS

115g (4oz/1 cup) dried goji berries
2 sweet potatoes, peeled
1 apple, peeled and grated
115g (4oz/1 cup) self-raising flour
2 eggs, separated
1 litre (35fl oz/4 cups) sunflower oil, for frying

Soak the goji berries in water. Chop the potatoes into 2.5cm (1in) cubes, boil for 10 minutes, drain and mash. Mix the mash, berries, apple, flour and egg yolks. Beat the egg whites until stiff and fold in. Deep-fry dollops in hot oil for 8–10 minutes. Drain and serve.

Runners often nibble on dried goji berries to boost energy levels that may be diminishing.

Research shows that exercise increases the need for anti-oxidants, so goji berries are a great choice for athletes because they're rich in phytonutrients with significant antioxidant properties. Goji berries are also one of the few fruit sources of omega-3 and -6 essential fatty acids, good for keeping joints oiled. They are rich in amino acids to help to improve stamina, and betaine, a complex phytonutrient used by the liver to produce choline – a compound that promotes muscle growth.

Goji berries are also sometimes known as wolf berries.

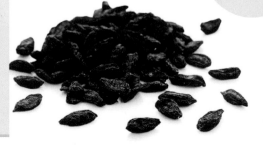

021

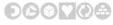

Blueberry

NUTRIENTS
Vitamins B2, C, E, beta-carotene, folic acid (folate); anthocyanins, ellagic acid, tannins; fibre

Popular in the US, these juicy berries get full marks for their health-giving properties.

Native to North America, blueberries have been used medicinally for centuries by Native North Americans, while members of the same plant family are known throughout the world for their healing abilities. They taste similar to blackcurrants, but without the sharpness. Blueberries are often stewed and sweetened, but for their full range of health benefits they are best eaten raw.

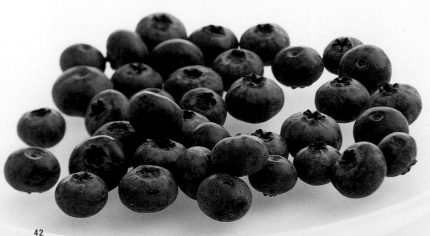

BLUEBERRIES' IMMUNITY-BOOSTING PROPERTIES

One serving of blueberries provides as many antioxidants as five servings of broccoli, apples or carrots, and studies have ranked them above all other fruit and vegetables for antioxidant activity. Ellagic acid, one of these antioxidants, is thought to prevent the development of cancer. Blueberries also contain the antioxidant anthocyanins, which strengthen blood capillaries, improving circulation and helping the transport of nutrients around the body – probably one of the reasons blueberries can enhance eyesight and protect against dementia, heart disease and strokes. They have an anti-inflammatory effect on the body's tissues, and are rich in tannins, which fight the bacteria that cause urinary tract infections.

USING BLUEBERRIES

Eat blueberries three or four times a week for full immunity-boosting benefits. They can be eaten raw as a snack, with plain bio-yogurt and nuts for a light breakfast, or combined with other berries and a little cream for a delicious dessert.

BLUEBERRY FACTS

• Native North Americans and early European settlers used blueberry root as a relaxant during childbirth. They also treated coughs with the juice and made tea from the leaves to help to purify the blood.

• Eating blueberries stains the tongue blue, owing to their health-giving anthocyanin pigment, which is water soluble.

• When cooked or dried much of the vitamin-C content in blueberries is destroyed, although they retain their flavonoid activity.

BLUEBERRY SMOOTHIE *serves 2–3*

250g (9oz/2 cups) blueberries
125g (4½oz/1 cup) raspberries
 or other summer berries
125ml (4fl oz/½ cup) plain
 bio-yogurt

Whizz everything together in a blender, then serve. When temperatures outside are sizzling, simply add four cubes of ice to the berries in the blender to make a cooling summer crush.

022

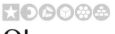

Cherry

NUTRIENTS
Vitamin C; potassium; anthocyanins, ellagic acid

These sweet summer treats are potent detoxifiers and are useful in the prevention of cancer.

Like many other berries, cherries contain ellagic acid – a powerful compound that blocks an enzyme that cancer cells need in order to develop. Cherries are also rich in anthocyanins, antioxidant substances that the body uses to help make disease-fighting chemicals, and they contain immune-essential vitamin C, and so can aid the fight against viruses and bacteria. In addition, they have anti-inflammatory properties, which ease rheumatoid arthritis and gout.

Infusions made from cherry stalks are a traditional remedy for cystitis.

CHOCO-CHERRIES

serves 2–4

200g (7oz) cherries, left on the stalk
100g (3½oz) good-quality plain/ bittersweet chocolate, melted

Dip each of the cherries into the chocolate. Place on a greased plate and chill until set.

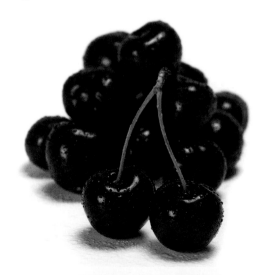

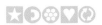

Passion Fruit

Dense with vitamins, this intensely fragrant fruit with edible seeds is an effective energy booster.

Passion fruit is a good source of vitamin C, which fights viruses and bacteria. It also contains carotenoids, which the body transforms into antioxidant vitamin A, an important cancer-fighter, while its B-vitamins help keep the muscles and nervous system healthy and maintain steady energy levels. In addition, passion fruit contains fibre, which is important for a healthy digestive system and heart.

Passion fruit contains substances which can help to ease depression and anxiety.

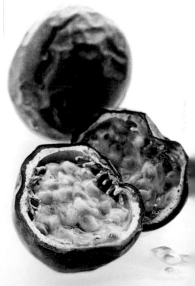

PASSION FRUIT SORBET *serves 4*

125g (4½oz/scant ⅔ cup) raw cane sugar
400ml (14fl oz/1¾ cups) passion fruit pulp, blended

Place the sugar in a large saucepan with 100ml (3½fl oz/ 7 tbsp) water and gently heat, stirring until the sugar dissolves. Bring to a boil, then reduce the heat and simmer for 1 minute. Remove from the heat and let cool. When cool, mix in the passion fruit. Place in a plastic container and freeze until solid. Stir before serving.

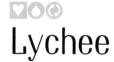

Lychee

NUTRIENTS
Vitamins B1, B2, C; copper, potassium

Light, rich in quick-energy carbohydrate and easily digestible, lychees make an exotic change from other fruit-bowl favourites.

Lychees are native to China, the Philippines and India.

Deliciously refreshing lychees are the perfect nutritious snack to have before exercise or between training sessions. Available fresh, dried or canned, nine lychees provide an adult's recommended daily intake of vitamin C and 15 per cent more polyphenols (which research shows help to keep the heart strong) than the equivalent number of grapes. To open a fresh lychee, score down one side with a sharp knife, peel off the crocodile-like skin and lift out the transparent, juicy flesh.

LYCHEE JELLY

8 lychees, peeled, pitted and halved
½ mango, peeled, pitted and cubed
55g (2oz/¼ cup) caster (superfine) sugar
2 x 11g (¼oz) sachets powdered gelatine
500ml (17fl oz/2 cups) apple juice

Place the lychees and mango in the bottom of 4 small jelly moulds or serving bowls. Heat the sugar in half the apple juice over a low heat until dissolved, then add the gelatine. Add the rest of the juice, pour over the fruit and refrigerate overnight. Tip out onto plates to serve.

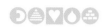

Grape

These sweet and juicy vine fruits are nature's cleansers and make excellent detoxifiers.

Grapes are rich in antioxidant anthocyanins, which help to strengthen capillaries, so they are an excellent food for helping to improve circulation and heart health. Their high antioxidant content means that they are helpful for mopping up harmful free radicals, making them powerful detoxifiers of the skin, liver, kidneys, and bowels. Grapes can help to stabilise immune response by moderating allergic reactions. They also contain cancer-preventing ellagic acid.

NUTRIENTS
Vitamins B3, B6, biotin; potassium, selenium, zinc; anthocyanins, ellagic acid

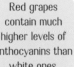

Red grapes contain much higher levels of anthocyanins than white ones.

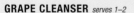

GRAPE CLEANSER *serves 1–2*

20 seedless grapes
6 stalks of celery
handful of watercress

Press the ingredients through a juicer, alternating the grapes, celery, and watercress. Mix well, and drink immediately.

Date

NUTRIENTS
Vitamins B3, B5, B6, C, K,
beta-carotene, folic acid (folate);
calcium, copper, iodine, iron,
magnesium, manganese, phosphorus,
potassium, selenium, zinc

Dates can be
frozen for up
to a year in an
airtight container.

**Chewy, dried dates make excellent "survival food"
on long bike rides or when hiking.**

The ideal preparation for exercise is to eat a light meal three hours
before you begin, and then to top up with a snack just half an hour
before. Dates are the perfect snack option – they're high in
carbohydrates for energy and an excellent source of potassium,
which is important for maintaining the fluid and electrolyte
balances in the body.

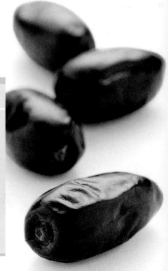

FRUIT SQUARES

115g (4oz/⅔ cup) dried dates
**115g (4oz/⅔ cup) dried
apricots**
125ml (4fl oz/½ cup) lime juice
**250g (9oz/2 cups) self-raising
flour**
**100g (3½oz/½ cup) caster
(granulated) sugar**
3 eggs, beaten

Blend the dates, apricots and
lime juice in a food processor.
Mix in the flour, sugar and eggs.
Spoon the mixture into a
greased 18cm (7in) square cake
pan. Bake in a pre-heated oven
at 180°C/350°F/Gas 4 for 30–35
minutes. Allow to cool, then cut
into squares.

Fig

Nature's own laxative, figs are indigenous to Persia, Syria and other parts of Asia, and are generously high in healthful compounds.

Figs contain active ingredients that stimulate the intestinal action needed for bowel movement. They are also a rich source of soluble fibre, which has a laxative effect.

Figs contain good amounts of potassium, a mineral that is essential for keeping blood pressure down. Being rich in iron, they are excellent for pregnant women and convalescents. Used topically, they are good at drawing out poisons.

PROPERTIES/ACTIONS
- Laxative
- High in fibre
- Rich in potassium

PARTS USED
- Whole fruit

FIG SYRUP
for constipation

50g (2oz/⅓ cup) dried figs
50g (2oz/⅓ cup) prunes
1 tbsp treacle

Put the figs and prunes in a saucepan with 455ml (16fl oz/ 2 cups) water. Soak for 8 hours, then bring to the boil and simmer until the fruit is soft and the excess liquid has reduced. Stir in the treacle, then cool and whizz in a food processor. Transfer to a jam jar and store in the refrigerator. Take 1 dessertspoon of the syrup as needed.

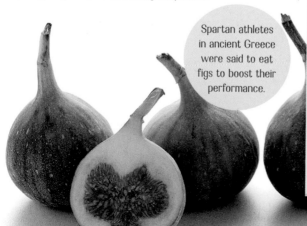

Spartan athletes in ancient Greece were said to eat figs to boost their performance.

Star Fruit

The exotic star fruit lives up to its name thanks to its powerful antioxidant properties.

Also known as the star apple or carambola, the star fruit is completely edible: as well as the small soft seeds found inside, the external skin can be washed and eaten, too.

BOOSTS IMMUNITY

Nutritionally, star fruit is a good source of disease-fighting beta-carotene. It is also packed with vitamin C, important for serious athletes because the body releases stress hormones into the bloodstream during heavy training, which can temporarily suppress the immune system. Eating vitamin-C-rich foods counteracts this by significantly raising antioxidant levels.

NUTRIENTS
Vitamin C, beta-carotene, folic acid (folate); potassium

STAR FRUIT FACTS
• The star fruit originates from Sri Lanka.

•Harvested when green, star fruit gradually turn a bright yellow, then a darker shade with brown tips when stored. This signals optimal ripeness, but doesn't impair texture or nutritional value.

•Anyone with kidney problems should avoid star fruit because of its oxalic acid content.

•In Chinese medicine, star fruit is known for its diuretic properties.

•In the Philippines, star fruit is eaten sprinkled with a little salt.

SWEET AND SOUR NOODLES

300g (10½oz) egg noodles
2 tbsp sesame oil
500g (1lb 2oz) cooked prawns
  (shrimp), shelled and deveined
4 small star fruit, sliced
  and tips removed
1 tbsp soy sauce
juice and zest of 1 lime

Cook the noodles according to the packet instructions, then drain. Meanwhile, heat the oil in a pan until hot. Add the prawns, star fruit, and soy sauce and stir-fry for 3 minutes. Toss with the noodles and lime juice and zest, and serve.

CORRECTS FLUID RETENTION

Star fruit also contains potassium, which has a mild diuretic effect, promoting the elimination of excess water.

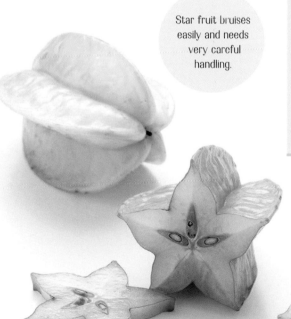

Star fruit bruises easily and needs very careful handling.

TROPICAL FLAPJACKS

175g (6oz/¾ cup) butter
100g (3½oz/½ cup) soft brown sugar
5 tbsp maple syrup
225g (8oz/2¼ cups) rolled oats
115g (4oz) dried star fruit pieces

Melt the butter, sugar and maple syrup in a pan, then mix in the oats and star fruit. Press the mixture into a greased 20cm (8in) baking tin and bake in a pre-heated oven at 180°C/350°F/Gas 4 for 25 minutes. Slice into squares when cool.

NATURE'S PHARMACY

Olive

NUTRIENTS
Vitamins E, K, beta-carotene; calcium, copper, iodine, iron, magnesium, manganese, phosphorus, potassium, selenium, zinc; omega-9 essential fatty acids

Staples of Mediterranean cuisine, olives are bursting with health benefits.

There are hundreds of olive varieties. In general, black varieties are moist and full flavoured, while green have a milder taste.

BEST FOR THE HEART
Olives are thought to keep the heart healthy because they're among the best sources of monounsaturated fats, which help to lower harmfully high cholesterol levels.

OLIVE FACTS
•The oil made from olives is one of the healthiest culinary oils as it contains lots of monounsaturates, which are good for the heart.

• Olive oil is available in a variety of grades, which reflect the degree to which it has been processed. "Extra virgin" is the best choice, as it retains the most antioxidants.

•Store olives and olive oils in opaque tubs and dark, tinted bottles, as these will help to prevent the harmful oxidation caused by exposure to light.

PROTECTS JOINTS
Super-rich in vitamin E and omega-9 fatty acids, which have anti-inflammatory properties, olives also help to protect the joints from

---

OLIVE AND NUT DIP

225g (8oz/2¼ cups) pitted green olives
100g (3½oz/¾ cup) shelled walnuts
55g (2oz/½ cup) pine nuts
2 tbsp grated Romano cheese
1 tbsp olive oil
breadsticks, to serve

Whizz the olives, walnuts and pine nuts in a blender until smooth. Mix in the grated cheese and olive oil. Serve with breadsticks.

workout wear and tear. In addition, the essential fatty acids in olives have been shown to boost the body's ability to remove unwanted stored fat in the cells.

STRENGTHENS BONES

One recent scientific study suggests that eating olives on a regular basis also plays an important role in protecting bones against osteoporosis.

MINI KEBABS *Makes 24*

24 black olives, pitted
 and halved
24 cherry tomatoes, halved
24 cubes feta cheese
48 basil leaves
black pepper

Spear 2 olive halves, 2 tomato halves, 2 basil leaves and a cube of cheese onto each of 24 cocktail sticks (toothpicks), alternating ingredients. Season, arrange on a serving dish and serve.

In the wild, olive trees bear fruit only every other year.

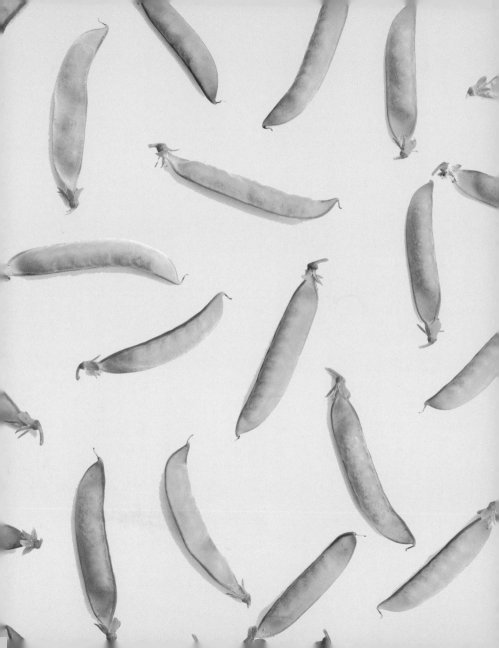

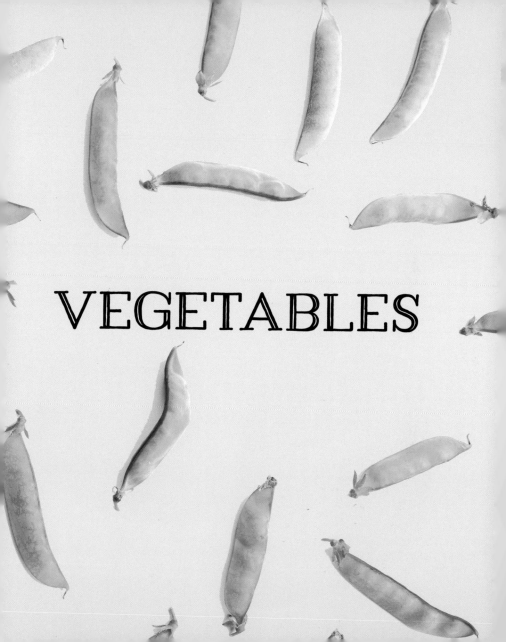

VEGETABLES

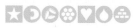

Avocado

NUTRIENTS
Vitamins B1, B2, B3, B5, E, K, biotin, carotenoids, folic acid (folate); potassium, zinc; beta-sitosterol, glutathione; omega-6 fatty acids; fibre

One of the few fruits that contains fat, avocado boasts a wealth of health-boosting properties.

Strictly speaking, avocado is a fruit, although it is typically used in savoury dishes. It is native to Central America, and was discovered by Spanish invaders in the 16th century. It is now popular throughout the world and grown in various tropical regions. With a smooth, buttery texture and mild, creamy taste, avocado is best eaten when ripe.

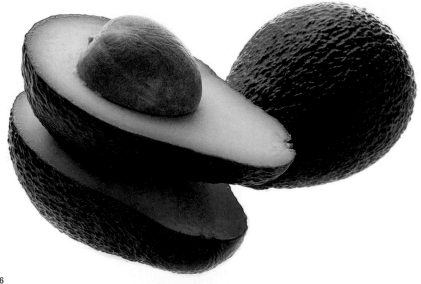

AVOCADO'S IMMUNITY-BOOSTING PROPERTIES

Avocados contains monounsaturated fat which can help to lower cholesterol. They are also a source of linoleic acid (known as omega-6 fatty acid), which the body converts to gamma-linolenic acid (GLA), a substance that helps to thin the blood, soothe inflammation and improve blood-sugar balance. They are rich in vitamin E, an antioxidant that neutralises the damaging effect of toxins in the body and boosts resistance to infection. Avocado's B-vitamin levels help the immune cells to destroy harmful invaders – as does glutathione, a powerful substance that boosts the action of the body's natural killer cells. Last but not least, they contain the plant chemical beta-sitosterol which is particularly beneficial to the prostate gland.

USING AVOCADO

Avocados are normally picked before they are ripe, and take about a week to ripen at room temperature, although storing them in a paper bag with a banana can speed the process.

AVOCADO FACTS

• The avocado has been known by several names, including alligator pear and butter pear. It earned the title butter pear because of its smooth texture, but alligator pear was the original name given to it by the Spanish.

• Stop opened avocados from turning brown by sprinkling the exposed surfaces with lemon juice and leaving the stone in.

• Avocado is also an effective skin treatment – simply mash the flesh and smooth it over your face, washing off after 10 minutes, to nourish your complexion.

• People with latex allergies are also likely to be allergic to avocado.

GUACAMOLE *makes 1 large bowl*

2 ripe avocados, peeled and pitted
juice of 1 lime
2 garlic cloves, crushed
1 medium onion, finely chopped
2 tomatoes, skinned and chopped

1 small red chilli, deseeded and finely chopped
1 tbsp finely chopped coriander (cilantro)

For a chunky dip, mash the avocados by hand with the lime juice until smooth, then add the remaining ingredients and combine thoroughly. For a smoother texture blend the ingredients in a food processor Serve as a dip for crudités.

⊙⊙🛡🔥

Spinach

NUTRIENTS

Vitamins B2, B3, C, E, carotenoids, folic acid (folate); calcium, magnesium, zinc; fibre

---

SPINACH RISOTTO   *serves 4*

1 tbsp olive oil
55g (2oz/¼ cup) unsalted butter
2 onions, finely chopped
275g (9½oz/1½ cups) Arborio rice
1 small glass white wine
850ml (29fl oz/3½ cups) vegetable stock
4 good handfuls fresh spinach
100g (3½oz/1½ cups) grated Parmesan cheese

Heat the oil and butter in a pan, and fry the onions until golden. Add the rice, stir for 1 minute, then add the wine and leave until absorbed. Add enough stock to cover, leave to absorb, and keep adding until all the stock is used and the rice is cooked. Stir in the spinach and cook until wilted. Remove from heat and sprinkle with cheese.

This versatile leafy vegetable is popular worldwide and has powerful anti-carcinogenic properties.

Spinach is rich in carotenoids, which the body converts to antioxidant vitamin A to help to trigger immune response to fight infections. This vegetable helps to prevent lung, breast and cervical cancers, as well as to fight heart disease. Its vitamin C content keeps skin and mucous membranes healthy, while its B vitamins improve energy and nervous-system conditions. Spinach is also rich in zinc, required to promote T-cell activity.

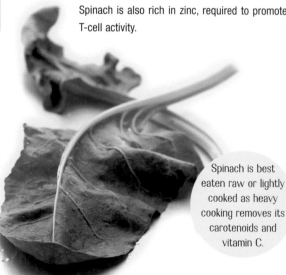

Spinach is best eaten raw or lightly cooked as heavy cooking removes its carotenoids and vitamin C.

Watercress

This robustly-flavoured salad leaf is a powerful immune system stimulant.

Watercress is rich in glucosinolates – plant chemicals that boost the activity of cancer-preventing enzymes. It contains the key antioxidant vitamins needed for a fully-functioning immune system, along with vitamin B6, which enhances the action of phagocytes – white blood cells responsible for cleaning up waste matter. Watercress is also a good source of the mineral manganese, and iron, which can both help the body to resist infections.

NUTRIENTS
Vitamins B3, B6, C, E, K, beta-carotene (and other carotenoids); calcium, manganese, iron, zinc; glucosinolates; fibre

WATERCRESS DIP
makes 1 bowl

large handful of watercress leaves, chopped
1 onion, chopped
1 ripe avocado, peeled, pitted and sliced
juice of ½ a lemon
pinch of vegetable bouillon powder
1 garlic clove

Place all the ingredients together in a blender and process until smooth. Serve as a dip for crudités.

Traditionally watercress has been used to boost the metabolism and detoxify the body.

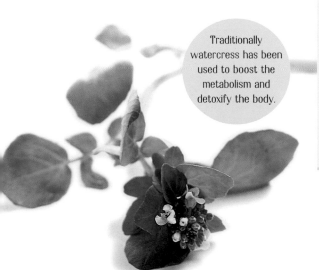

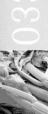

Celery

PROPERTIES/ACTIONS
- Stimulates kidneys
- Nervine
- Sedative

PARTS USED
- Whole vegetable

With its roots in 16th-century Italy, celery, a member of the parsley family, can stimulate the kidneys and help flush out the system.

Celery is good at aiding the elimination of waste via the urine, thus acting as a detoxifying agent. It is an anti-inflammatory, clearing uric acid from painful joints, and is well known as a remedy for gout and rheumatism. Celery is a useful antiseptic in the urinary tract and may help to lower blood pressure and prevent cancer. Celery seeds are more potent than other parts of the plant.

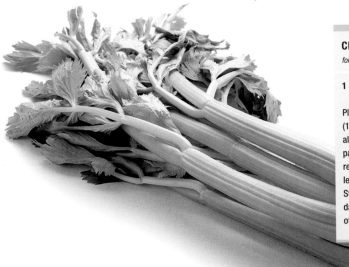

CELERY SEED TEA
for rheumatism & urinary infections

1 heaped tsp celery seeds

Place the seeds and 500ml (17fl oz/2 cups) water in an aluminium or a stainless steel pan. Bring to the boil, then remove from the heat and leave to infuse for 10 minutes. Strain. Drink up to 3 times a day depending on the severity of symptoms.

Lettuce

Vitamins B1, B3, B5, C, E, K, beta-carotene, folic acid (folate); calcium, iodine, iron, magnesium, manganese, phosphorus, potassium, selenium, silica, zinc

CHEESY GRILLED LETTUCE

1 Romaine lettuce
1 tbsp olive oil
200g (7oz) Camembert
2 tsp balsamic vinegar

Cut the lettuce lengthways into quarters, brush with the oil and grill (broil) for 2 minutes on each side. Arrange in a shallow ovenproof dish, top with thin slices of cheese and drizzle over the vinegar. Bake in a pre-heated oven at 220°C/425°F/Gas 7 for 5 minutes until the cheese is bubbling, then serve.

A salad and sandwich staple, lettuce provides vital nutrients for helping the body to make energy.

Lettuce contains many minerals, including iron, calcium, magnesium and zinc, all of which help to generate energy. Equally important for health is the folic acid (folate) content – this B-vitamin protects the heart by converting a damaging chemical called homocysteine into benign substances. If not converted, homocysteine can directly damage blood vessels, greatly increasing the risk of heart attack and stroke.

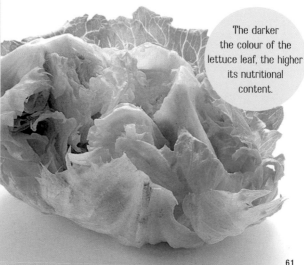

The darker the colour of the lettuce leaf, the higher its nutritional content.

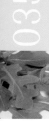

Rocket

This hot, peppery salad leaf is packed with essential disease-fighting nutrients.

NUTRIENTS

Vitamin C, beta-carotene; volatile oils; fibre; sulphoraphane

Rocket (arugula) contains high levels of vitamin C, a powerfully antioxidant nutrient that helps to prevent the body against toxins and boosts resistance to viruses and other infections. It is also rich in beta-carotene, which the body uses to make cancer-fighting vitamin A. Rocket contains high concentrations of sulphoraphane, a substance shown to have potent anti-cancer properties, and it is a good source of fibre.

ROCKET AND STEAK OPEN SANDWICHES *serves 4*

4 slices wholegrain bread
150g (5½oz/⅔ cup) butter
2 tbsp chopped parsley
4 minute steaks
2 large tomatoes, sliced
large handful of rocket
(arugula) leaves, washed

Lightly toast the bread on both sides. Mix together the butter and parsley, and spread over the toast. Grill (broil) the steaks for 1 minute on each side, then place them on top of the toast slices. Top with the tomatoes and rocket leaves and serve.

Rocket can be cooked lightly, but it is more frequently used raw, as a salad vegetable.

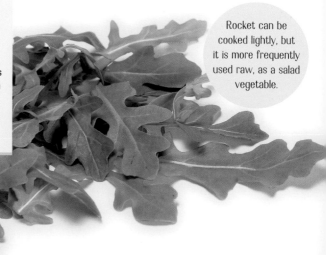

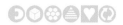

Belgian Endive

NUTRIENTS
Vitamins B1, folic acid (folate), beta-carotene; iron, phosphorous; fibre

A good digestive stimulant, endive was originally grown for its root which was added to coffee.

Belgian endive (also known as chicory) contains bitters, which help to stimulate the digestive system and detoxify the liver. It is also rich in beta-carotene, which is converted by the body into vitamin A – an antioxidant that helps to prevent cancer and has potent anti-viral properties. It also contains vitamin B1, an important energy-booster that keeps mucous membranes and nerves healthy. Belgian endive is a good source of fibre, helping to regulate the elimination of waste from the body, and lowering cholesterol levels.

BRAISED ENDIVE *serves 2–3*

2 Belgian endives, sliced
1 small red apple, diced
2 tbsp lemon juice
2 tsp olive oil
2 tbsp white wine vinegar
1 tbsp parsley, chopped
sea salt and black pepper

Place all the ingredients, apart from the vinegar and the parsley, in a large saucepan and just cover with water. Cook on a low heat until the water evaporates. Drain, and sprinkle with the vinegar and the parsley, and season with salt and pepper to taste. Serve as a side dish.

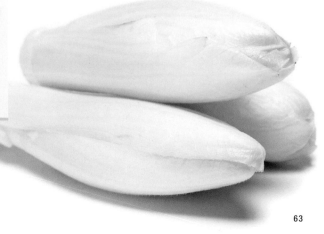

037

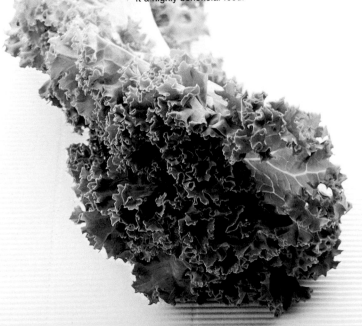

Curly Kale

NUTRIENTS

Vitamins B2, B3, B6, C, E, K, beta-carotene, folic acid (folate); calcium, iron, magnesium, zinc; flavonoids, glucosinolates, fibre

Bursting with vitamins and phytochemicals, kale is an important immunity-booster.

Curly kale is thought to have originated in the Mediterranean region. Like cabbage and Brussels sprouts, it is a member of the *Cruciferous* family, sharing with these vegetables the ability to retain high levels of water and nutrients in its leaves, which makes it a highly beneficial food.

CURLY KALE'S IMMUNITY-BOOSTING PROPERTIES

Kale contains high levels of glucosinolates, natural plant chemicals which block cancer-causing substances, stimulate detoxifying and repair enzymes in the body and suppress cancer cell division. It also contains flavonoids, which are needed for healthy circulation and to stimulate immune response, and plant sterols, important for keeping cholesterol levels low. In addition, curly kale is packed with B-vitamins that improve energy and bolster the immune system's ability to mop up invader cells. It has high levels of antioxidant vitamin C and beta-carotene. It also contains vitamin K, which promotes blood clotting and healing, and good amounts of immunity-boosting minerals, including iron and zinc.

USING CURLY KALE

Curly kale can be eaten raw, steamed and served as a side dish, or lightly stir-fried. Kale is in season in winter, and is a nutritious addition to the diet during the colder months.

CURLY KALE FACTS

• Curly kale, like other members of the Cruciferous family is thought to have hormone-balancing properties that help to prevent breast and ovarian cancer.

• Vegetables in the Cruciferous family are possibly the most important plant foods with regard to cancer prevention, because of their high glucosinolate content

• In some parts of Europe, curly kale is known as borecole, derived from a Dutch word meaning "peasants' cabbage".

• The nutrients in curly kale are particularly beneficial to the skin and encourage wound healing and maintenance of healthy cell membranes.

TENDER PARSLEY KALE *serves 4*

1kg (2lb 4oz) curly kale 2 tbsp olive oil 3 tbsp chopped parsley ½ tsp ground nutmeg sea salt and black pepper	Wash and shred the kale leaves. Heat the oil in a large saucepan, add the kale, cover and cook on a low heat until the leaves are tender. Season with salt and pepper, stir the parsley and nutmeg through for 1 minute, then serve immediately.

Savoy Cabbage

This tender leaf is a powerful detoxifier.

NUTRIENTS

Vitamins B3, C, folic acid (folate), beta-carotene; calcium, iron, potassium; glucosinolates; fibre

Savoy cabbage contains antioxidant vitamin C, needed for good overall immune function, and beta-carotene, which is converted into cancer-preventing vitamin A in the body. It is also a good source of vitamin B3 – needed for energy, and healthy muscles and nerves – and folic acid (folate), a key substance for good reproductive health. Savoy cabbage contains glucosinolates, plant chemicals containing powerful enzymes that research suggests help to protect against cancer.

SWEET SAVOY CABBAGE

serves 4

3 tbsp olive oil
1 tbsp mustard seeds
1 Savoy cabbage, shredded
2 garlic cloves, crushed
2 tbsp dessicated (dried shredded) coconut
1 tbsp maple syrup
2 tbsp lemon juice
sea salt and black pepper

Heat the oil in a wok, add the mustard seeds and stir-fry until they pop. Add the cabbage and garlic and fry until the leaves wilt, then add the coconut, maple syrup and lemon juice. Stir-fry for 1 minute and season. Serve as a side dish.

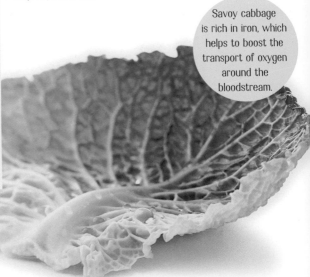

Savoy cabbage is rich in iron, which helps to boost the transport of oxygen around the bloodstream.

039

Brussels Sprouts

This relative of the cabbage is an effective cancer-fighter thanks to its high levels of antioxidants.

Brussels sprouts are one of the best sources of glucosinolates, which help the body to produce cancer-preventing enzymes. They are high in vitamin C and folic acid (folate), which encourage the body to heal itself. Brussels sprouts also contain vitamin B5, an immune stimulant that triggers the production of antibodies. Dense in fibre, Brussels sprouts keep the digestive system healthy and cholesterol low.

Brussels sprouts are named after the capital of Belgium, where they were first grown in the 16th century.

NUTRIENTS
Vitamins B2, B5, B6, C, folic acid (folate), beta-carotene; potassium; glucosinolates; fibre

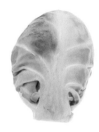

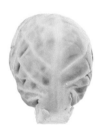

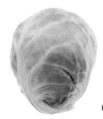

NUTTY SPROUT STIR-FRY *serves 4*

2 onions, peeled and sliced
150g (5½oz/1¼ cups) blanched
   almonds, lightly toasted
4 tbsp olive oil
600g (1lb 5oz) Brussels sprouts,
   peeled and sliced
sea salt and black pepper

Gently fry the onions and almonds in the oil until the onions are soft. Blanch the sprouts for 1 minute in a saucepan of lightly salted boiling water, then add to the pan with the onions and almonds, cooking gently until tender. Season to taste and serve.

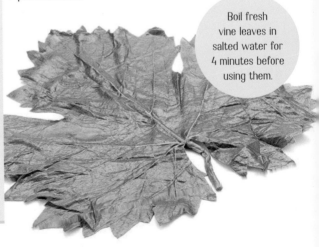

Vine Leaves

NUTRIENTS

Vitamin C, E, K; calcium, iron, magnesium, manganese, phosphorus, potassium, selenium, sodium, zinc

Commonly used in Greek cuisine, vine leaves contain flavonoid antioxidants to help to prevent post-exercise muscle soreness.

Tender, dark green vine leaves, with a subtle flavour and texture similar to spinach, are available fresh and ready-to-use in salt-water pouches. Like all leafy green vegetables, they contain flavonoids and vitamin C, useful for anyone working out regularly because a diet rich in antioxidants has been shown to promote faster recovery after exercise and to help the body stay in peak condition.

Boil fresh vine leaves in salted water for 4 minutes before using them.

STUFFED VINE LEAVES

400g (14oz) minced lamb
200g (7oz/1 cup) long-grain rice
handful of mint, chopped
1 tbsp olive oil
3 spring onions (scallions),
   finely chopped
16 vine leaves
sea salt and black pepper

Mix the lamb, rice, mint, oil and spring onions in a bowl, and season. Place 2 vine leaves on top of each other, add a dollop of the mixture and roll up to form a parcel. Repeat to make 8 parcels and place in a steamer over a pan of simmering water. Steam for 1 hour or until the leaves are tender, and the meat and rice are cooked. Serve 2 parcels each as a starter.

Chard

Eaten raw or cooked like spinach, chard is a valuable source of iron for those who enjoy a plant-based diet.

A member of the beet family, chard has crunchy stalks and spinach-like leaves with a slightly bitter, earthy flavour. Chard is an excellent bone-builder thanks to its calcium, magnesium and vitamin-K content, which are all thought to aid bone mineralization. Many of the nutrients in chard keep blood vessels strong, allowing blood to move oxygen around the body easily to boost strength and energy levels.

NUTRIENTS
Vitamins C, K, beta-carotene, folic acid (folate); calcium, iron, magnesium, zinc

CHARD WITH SESAME SEEDS

1 onion, finely chopped
1 tbsp olive oil
1 tbsp tamari sauce
55g (2oz/⅓ cup) sesame seeds
300g (10½oz) chard leaves

In a pan, fry the onion in the oil until soft. Stir in the tamari sauce and sesame seeds. Chop the chard leaves into slices, add to the pan and stir until wilted. Serve immediately.

Pak Choi

Crank up the nutritional content of stir-fries and spring rolls with this potent Chinese vegetable.

NUTRIENTS
Vitamins B2, B6, C, beta-carotene, folic acid (folate); calcium, iron, magnesium, manganese, phosphorus, potassium, selenium, zinc

Pak choi (bok choy) belongs to the cabbage family and has a mild, mustardy taste. Both the leaves and stalks are edible and packed with nutrients. Baby leaves with very fine stalks work brilliantly in salads. One average portion of cooked pak choi contains the same amount of calcium as 125ml (4fl oz/½ cup) of full-fat milk. Pak choi also has an abundance of vitamin C, which aids recovery from sports injuries by strengthening cell walls.

CRUNCHY VEGETABLE STIR-FRY

1 tbsp sesame oil
1 onion, finely chopped
1 garlic clove, crushed
½ cabbage, shredded
150g (5½oz) mushrooms, sliced
4 pak choi (bok choy) stalks, shredded

Heat the oil in a wok over a high heat. Add the onion and garlic and stir-fry for 2 minutes. Add the cabbage, mushrooms and pak choi and stir-fry for a further 4 minutes. Serve immediately.

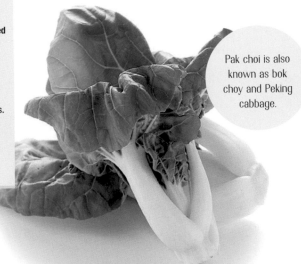

Pak choi is also known as bok choy and Peking cabbage.

Broccoli

A member of the cabbage family, broccoli has ancient beginnings. It has been shown to aid treatment of many conditions, including cancer.

Broccoli contains a number of chemical compounds, including indoles, carotenoids and the vitamin A precursor beta-carotene, known to inhibit the activation of cancer cells.

High in antioxidants, including vitamin C, broccoli is known to help boost immunity and prevent conditions such as heart disease and osteoporosis. It is rich in iron and therefore helps to treat anaemia, and is a good source of fibre.

PROPERTIES/ACTIONS
- Anti-cancer
- Boosts immunity

PARTS USED
- Vegetable head

WARM BROCCOLI & SESAME SALAD

1 head broccoli florets
2 tbsp olive oil
60ml (2fl oz/¼ cup) soy sauce
60ml (2fl oz/¼ cup) rice wine
    vinegar
2 tbsp sesame oil
4 tbsp sosame seeds, toasted

Preheat the oven to 200°C/
400°F/Gas 6. Blanch the
broccoli for 1 minute. Drain,
spread on a baking tray and
coat with olive oil. Roast for
10 minutes. Transfer to a bowl.
Combine the soy sauce, vinegar
and sesame oil. Stir in 3 tbsp
sesame seeds. Pour over the
broccoli. Sprinkle with the
remaining seeds.

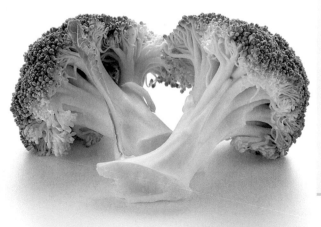

Pea

NUTRIENTS

Vitamins B-complex, C, K, beta-carotene, folic acid (folate); copper, iron, magnesium, manganese, phosphorus, potassium, zinc

PEA RISOTTO

1 onion, finely chopped
1 tbsp olive oil
300g (10½oz/2 cups) peas
175g (6oz/¾ cup) Arborio rice
250ml (9fl oz/1 cup) milk
750ml (26fl oz/3 cups) hot vegetable stock
handful of mint, chopped
55g (2oz/¾ cup) grated Parmesan cheese

In a heavy-bottomed pan, fry the onion in the oil until soft. Add the peas and cook for 2 minutes. Stir in the rice and milk. Gradually add the stock one ladle at a time, stirring until absorbed. Cook for 20 minutes. Then, gently stir in the mint, sprinkle the cheese over the top and serve.

For the weight conscious, peas are an excellent, quick-to-cook side dish.

Exceptionally rich in both soluble and insoluble fibre, peas are one of nature's best aids to weight control. Studies demonstrate that the more fibre we consume, the less likely we are to gain weight and the more readily we shed excess fat. Fibre has also been shown to have a positive effect on the hormones in the intestines that control appetite. In addition, the vitamin C and iron in peas help to keep energy levels topped up.

An average portion of frozen peas contains the same amount of vitamin C as two large apples.

Green Bean

Crunchy green beans are rich in disease-fighting vitamins and minerals.

Like other pulses, green beans are low in fat and high in soluble fibre, which is important for a healthy heart. They have high levels of B-vitamins, needed for the development of phagocyte cells, which mop up unwanted invaders, and also contain beta-carotene, which the body converts to cancer-preventing vitamin A. Green beans are also a good source of manganese, needed for the production of the anti-viral substance interferon.

Choose fresh, firm green beans as these contain the highest levels of nutrients.

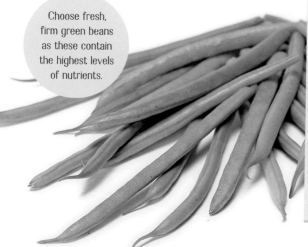

NUTRIENTS
Vitamins B3, folic acid (folate), beta-carotene; iron, manganese; fibre

BEAN AND RICE SALAD
serves 4

250g (9oz/1¼ cups) Arborio rice, cooked and cooled
150g (5½oz) green beans
1 bunch of asparagus, cut into small pieces
200g (7oz) canned kidney beans, drained
1 red (bell) pepper, chopped
20 green olives, pitted and halved
3 tbsp chopped parsley
3 tbsp chopped mint
5 spring onions (scallions), chopped
3 tbsp white wine vinegar
2 tbsp olive oil

Steam the green beans and asparagus until al dente. Allow to cool, then place in a bowl with the rice. Add the remaining ingredients and mix well. Leave to stand for 1 hour, then serve.

NATURE'S PHARMACY

Mangetout

NUTRIENTS
Vitamins B1, B2, B3, B5, C, beta-carotene, biotin; calcium, iron; fibre

These young pea pods have a delicate, sweet flavour as well as many health benefits.

High in B-vitamins, mangetout (snow peas) help to maintain energy levels and build nerve and muscle tissue. They contain immunity-stimulant vitamin B5, and antioxidant vitamin C. Mangetout are also a good source of fibre, which helps lower cholesterol levels and promote an efficient digestive system.

MANGETOUT STIR-FRY
serves 4

2 tbsp sesame oil
600g (1lb 5oz) firm tofu, cubed
25g (1oz/2 tbsp) butter
2 garlic cloves, crushed
2 red chillies, deseeded and
** finely chopped**
2 tsp grated fresh ginger,
750g (1lb 10oz) mangetout
** (snow peas)**
2 tbsp soy sauce

In a wok, heat half the oil, then stir-fry the tofu until browned. Set aside. Add the remaining oil and butter to the wok, then stir-fry the garlic, chilli and ginger. Add the peas, stir-frying until tender. Return the tofu to the wok, combine thoroughly, add the soy sauce and serve.

Mangetout are eaten whole and valued for their pods, rather than their peas.

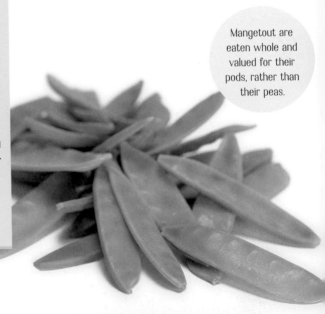

Asparagus

In mythology asparagus has been renowned since ancient times both as an aphrodisiac and medicinally, for its healing properties.

With its active compound asparagine stimulating the kidneys, bladder and liver, asparagus is a powerful diuretic. Its anti-inflammatory action helps treat rheumatoid arthritis and its high fibre content inhibits bacterial growth in the intestines, thus staving off conditions such as irritable bowel syndrome.

Asparagus is an excellent source of folic acid (folate), which is said to prevent birth defects. It also contains various antioxidants to fight cancerous cells and cardiovascular disease.

Ancient Egyptian tomb drawings suggest that asparagus was grown in 4000BCE.

PROPERTIES/ACTIONS
- Diuretic
- Stimulating

PARTS USED
- Asparagus spears

ASPARAGUS TINCTURE
for inflammatory conditions

10 young asparagus spears
500ml (17fl oz/2 cups) vodka

Chop the asparagus and place in a glass jar. Immerse in vodka and seal the jar tightly. Stand in a dark, cool place for 10 days, then discard the asparagus. Take 8–10 drops with 1 tbsp water 3 times a day, as needed.

048

Aubergine

Thanks to its high number of healing compounds, aubergine helps to ward off many illnesses.

NUTRIENTS
Vitamins B1, B3, B6, C, K, beta-carotene, folic acid (folate); calcium, copper, iodine, iron, magnesium, manganese, phosphorus, potassium, selenium, zinc

Aubergines (eggplants) are loaded with antioxidants, including chlorogenic acid, which is anti-viral, anti-bacterial and anti-fungal, and nasunin, a flavonoid found to mop up free radicals, protecting the body against diseases. A member of the nightshade family, aubergines should be avoided by sufferers of osteoarthritis as they may increase inflammation in the joints.

AUBERGINE AND RICOTTA ROLLS

1 large aubergine (eggplant),
    ends trimmed
3 tbsp olive oil
juice and zest of 1 lemon
200g (7oz) ricotta cheese
4 sun-dried tomatoes, chopped
black pepper

Cut the aubergine lengthways into 5mm (¼in) thick slices.

Cover with the oil and lemon juice and zest. Place on a baking tray and grill (broil) for 3 minutes on each side. Put some cheese, tomato and black pepper on each slice. Fold and secure with a cocktail stick (toothpick). Grill for a further 2 minutes, then serve.

Tomato

A favourite ingredient in many dishes, this juicy, sumptuous fruit was discovered by the early Aztecs of South America and is recognized today for its cancer-preventing nutrients.

Tomatoes are filled with the antioxidant vitamins C and E, as well as beta-carotene. They can help to prevent everything from cataracts to heart disease and cancer.

Lycopene, which gives tomatoes their vivid red colour, may also lower the risk of cancer, particularly cancer of the prostate, breast, lung and endometrium. This nutrient additionally helps people to stay active for longer.

PROPERTIES/ACTIONS
- Boots immunity
- Fights cancer

PARTS USED
- Whole tomato

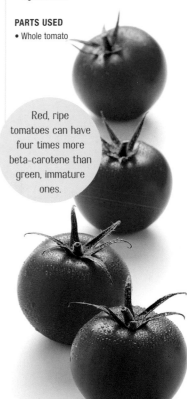

Red, ripe tomatoes can have four times more beta-carotene than green, immature ones.

SUN-DRIED TOMATO PESTO

24 sun-dried tomatoes, pre-soaked in oil
75g (3oz/⅗ cup) macadamia nuts, chopped
150g (5½oz/5 cups) basil leaves
3 garlic cloves, crushed
½ tbsp tomato purée (paste)
1½ tbsp balsamic vinegar
1 tbsp lemon juice

250ml (9fl oz/1 cup) tomato juice
4 tbsp olive oil
sea salt and black pepper

Blend all the ingredients together in a food processor until smooth. Transfer to a bowl and season to taste. Store for up to 5 days in the refrigerator.

Artichoke

PROPERTIES/ACTIONS
- Protects liver
- Supports gallbladder

PARTS USED
- Leaves & heart

Recognized mostly for its detoxifying effects, globe artichoke protects the liver and supports the gallbladder, making it a useful vegetable in many traditional remedies.

Originating in the Mediterranean, artichokes are the unopened flower buds of a thistle-like perennial plant. Each bud consists of several parts: overlapping outer leaves that are tough and inedible at the tip, but fleshy and tender at the base; an inedible choke, or thistle, which is enclosed within a light-coloured cone of immature leaves; and a round, firm-fleshed base, known as the heart. Collectively, artichokes contain vitamin C, high levels of B vitamins, dietary fibre, and a multitude of minerals. Both the leaves and heart have a long history of therapeutic use.

Containing an active ingredient called cynarin, artichokes, particularly the leaves, can help the liver to cope with an onslaught of rich party food and excess alcohol by maintaining a steady flow of bile – a fluid that helps the body to digest fats. Since artichokes are also a rich source of energy, taking the tincture is a great way to help to cure a hangover.

Because of their detoxifying qualities, artichokes are also a useful addition to the diet of people suffering from conditions like gout, arthritis and rheumatism. Traditionally, artichokes have been used to help to control blood cholesterol and to lower blood sugar.

ARTICHOKE TINCTURE

**150g (5½oz/5½ cups) dried artichoke leaves
300ml (10fl oz/1¼ cups) alcohol, preferably vodka**

Remove the leaves. Dry them individually, then grind them as finely as possible. Place the ground leaves in a glass jar. Cover with the alcohol and then with 600ml (20fl oz/2½ cups) water. Seal the jar tightly and leave in a dark, cool place for 2 weeks, shaking daily. Strain the liquid through a muslin (cheesecloth) into a dark glass bottle. Take 5–30 drops three times a day, as needed.

The hearts are particularly good for helping to combat indigestion if eaten at the beginning of a meal.

Make sure you wash artichokes thoroughly as dirt often gets between the leaves.

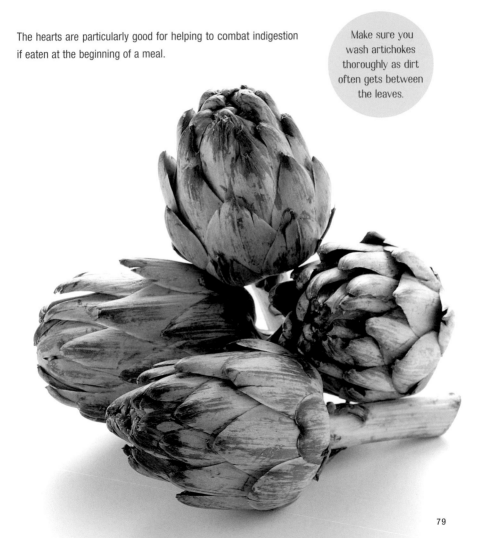

Sweetcorn

Barbecued or boiled, sweetcorn is a crunchy and deliciously sweet accompaniment to meat.

NUTRIENTS

Vitamins B3, B5, C, beta-carotene, folic acid (folate); magnesium, phosphorus, potassium, zinc

SWEETCORN RELISH

2 corn on the cob
55g (2oz/4 tbsp) butter
1 red (bell) pepper, deseeded and finely diced
1 red onion, finely diced
2 celery stalks, finely diced
½ cucumber, finely diced

Boil the corn in a large pan of salted water for 7–8 minutes until tender. Drain, slice off the kernels and mix with the butter. Mix well with the remaining ingredients.

Sweetcorn, made up of the yellow or white kernels that grow on the cob, is the most nutritious way to eat corn, as it provides starchy carbohydrates and a vegetable source of protein for a steady stream of energy during exercise. Yellow sweetcorn is a good source of the potent antioxidant lutein, which promotes healthy vision and a strong cardiovascular system. When canned or frozen, sweetcorn retains most of its goodness.

To stop corn burning on a barbecue, soak it in water for 10 minutes and wrap in foil before cooking.

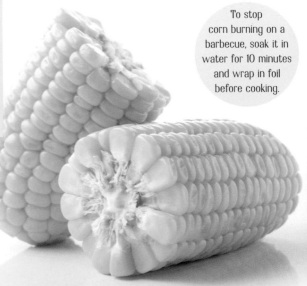

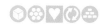

Red Pepper

Brightly coloured capsicum peppers are bursting with vitamin C and beta-carotene.

Red (bell) peppers are one of the best sources of vitamin C, which is crucial for immune function. They also contain flavonoids that are thought to enhance vitamin C's antioxidant action by strengthening its ability to protect the body against disease. Peppers have high levels of beta-carotene, which the body turns into anti-viral, immunity-boosting vitamin A, and also contain fibre, which is important for preventing the build up of cholesterol.

NUTRIENTS
Vitamins B6, C, beta-carotene; fibre

STUFFED PEPPERS *serves 4*

3 tbsp olive oil
200g (7oz) cherry tomatoes
2 garlic cloves, finely chopped
1 red onion, finely chopped
1 bunch basil, shredded
100g (3½oz) mozzarella cheese, cut into small cubes
100g (3½oz/1½ cups) grated Parmesan cheese
4 red (bell) peppers, topped and deseeded
black pepper

Preheat the oven to 220°C/425°F/Gas 7. Spoon 2 tbsp olive oil into an ovenproof dish and place in the oven. Meanwhile, combine all the ingredients except the peppers in a bowl with 1 tbsp olive oil. Fill each pepper with equal amounts of the mixture, then put the tops on. Place in the dish and bake for 20 minutes. Serve immediately.

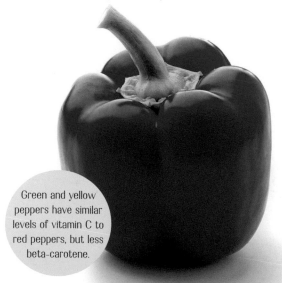

Green and yellow peppers have similar levels of vitamin C to red peppers, but less beta-carotene.

Beetroot

NUTRIENTS
Folic acid (folate); iron, manganese, potassium; betanin; fibre, protein

A useful detoxifier and blood purifier, beetroot is rich in a variety of nutrients crucial for immunity.

A descendant of the sea beet, which grows around the Mediterranean coast, beetroot (beet) has long been prized for its medicinal qualities. Traditionally, it has been used for purifying the blood. It is thought that beetroot was first used in Roman times and then introduced as a cooking ingredient by French chefs in the 18th century, when they began using it in dishes.

BEETROOT'S IMMUNITY-BOOSTING PROPERTIES

Rich in iron, beetroot enhances the production of disease-fighting antibodies, white blood cells (including phagocytes). It also stimulates red blood cells and improves the supply of oxygen to cells. It contains manganese, which is needed for the formation of interferon, a powerful anti-cancer substance, and is given its red colour by the pigment betanin, an antioxidant anthocyanin which can help prevent cancer and heart disease. Beetroot is thought to have detoxifying properties which improve liver and kidney health, and is high in fibre, important for both heart and digestive health.

USING BEETROOT

As effective cooked as it is raw, fresh beetroot can be juiced, used in salads or made into soup. Beetroot tops (leaves) are also rich in vitamin A and C, iron and calcium and can be used in a similar way to spinach. Simply boil them for a few minutes and serve warm with a little olive oil.

BEETROOT FACTS

• Beetroot was prized by the ancient Greeks, who would offer it up to their gods.

• Although beetroot contains no potential toxins, its tops (leaves) are high in oxalic acid, so they should be avoided by anyone with arthritis or kidney stones.

• Beetroot has traditionally been used by herbalists as a remedy for blood ailments and it is still considered to be an effective, naturopathic treatment in modern times.

• Betanin, the pigment that produces the red colouring in beetroot, can turn urine pink. This may be alarming but it is harmless!

HOT BEET SOUP *serves 2*

1 onion, peeled and chopped
1 garlic clove, crushed
1 tsp chilli powder
1 tbsp olive oil
400g (14oz) canned tomatoes
2 fresh beetroots (beets), washed
sour cream, to serve

Preheat the oven to 200°C/400°F/ Gas 6. Wrap each beetroot in foil and bake for about 45 minutes until tender. Leave them to cool, then peel and dice. Sweat the garlic and onions over a low heat in the olive oil for 3 minutes. Add the chilli powder, stir together for 1 minute, add the tomatoes and bring to the boil. Simmer for 15 minutes before stirring in the beetroot. Pour the soup into bowls, add some sour cream and serve.

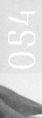

054

Pumpkin

NUTRIENTS
Vitamin C, beta-carotene; fibre

The most famous of all the winter squashes has flesh crammed with cancer-fighting chemicals.

Orange-fleshed pumpkins contain high levels of carotenoids, which studies suggest may help to prevent some forms of cancer – including cancer of the colon – as well as heart disease. Pumpkins are also rich in antioxidant vitamin C, which is needed for efficient immune system function, and can help to fight viruses such as colds, and improve general overall resistance to disease. In addition, pumpkins contain fibre, which helps to lower cholesterol, and promotes good digestion by encouraging the elimination of waste.

Choose orange pumpkins as they contain the highest amount of carotenoids.

PUMPKIN FRITTERS *serves 2*

1 medium pumpkin, cut into
    thick slices
175g (6oz/1⅓ cups) wholemeal
    flour
½ tsp salt
½ tsp baking powder
2 tsp ground cumin
1 egg, separated
1 onion, chopped

2 garlic cloves, crushed
2 tbsp olive oil

Steam the pumpkin for 10 minutes, then leave to cool. In a bowl, combine the flour, salt, baking powder and cumin, then add the egg yolk. Add 175ml (6fl oz/¾ cup) water, a little at

a time, stirring to form a smooth paste. Add the onion and garlic, then whisk the egg white and fold it in to the mixture. Heat the oil in a frying pan, then dip the pumpkin slices in the mixture and fry a few at a time, turning regularly, until crisp and brown. Serve warm.

Carrot

Carrots are packed with nutrients, which are particularly beneficial for eye health and vision.

Carrots are one of the richest sources of beta-carotene, which is converted by the body into the antioxidant vitamin A. This helps to strengthen cells against viruses, to fight cancer and to prevent heart disease. It also aids vision. We use the vitamin K present in carrots for bloodclotting and the healing of wounds, while their fibre content aids digestion and keeps the heart healthy. The chromium found in carrots helps to stabilise blood sugar levels, making this vegetable useful for controlling diabetes and sugar cravings.

NUTRIENTS
Vitamin K, beta-carotene, folic acid (folate); calcium, chromium, iron, zinc; fibre

ZINGY CARROT JUICE
serves 2

8 carrots, scrubbed and sliced
4 green apples, sliced
5cm (2in) piece fresh ginger

Press all the ingredients through a juicer. Serve immediately.

Raw carrots can be hard to digest, so grate or chop them finely before eating.

Butternut Squash

NUTRIENTS

Vitamins B1, B3, B5, B6, C, E, K, beta-carotene, folic acid (folate); calcium, copper, iron, magnesium, phosphorus, potassium, selenium, zinc

Squash is a nutritional winner and is delicious in soups and stews and with other roasted vegetables.

BOOSTS IMMUNITY

Like all orange fruit and vegetables, the butternut squash is a great source of beta-carotene, which the body converts to vitamin A, needed for a healthy immune system and good digestive and respiratory-tract function.

> You can tell if a squash is ripe by tapping it – if ripe, it will sound hollow.

SPICY ROASTED VEGETABLES

3 tbsp sunflower seeds
1 tsp chilli powder
1 tsp cumin seeds
1 tsp ground coriander
1 tsp ground ginger
1 butternut squash, peeled
   and deseeded
2 courgettes (zucchini), chopped
1 red (bell) pepper, deseeded
   and sliced
200g (7oz) button mushrooms
3 tbsp olive oil
1 tbsp balsamic vinegar

Toast the sunflower seeds and spices in a frying pan over a low heat for 3 minutes. Chop the squash into 5cm (2in) chunks. Place the squash and the other vegetables in an ovenproof dish. Add the oil, balsamic vinegar, seeds and spices, and mix well together. Bake in a pre-heated oven at 190°C/375°F/Gas 5 for 1 hour, stirring occasionally, then serve.

SUSTAINS ENERGY

A great provider of energy-sustaining carbohydrates, squash contains high levels of the minerals potassium and magnesium, which help to maintain efficient energy production. A lack of these minerals can lead to fatigue, muscle cramps and an increased risk of high cholesterol, high blood pressure and heart problems. Squashes are also thought to reduce the symptoms of prostatic hyperplasia, a benign prostate condition.

BUTTERNUT SQUASH FACTS

• Archaeologists have found evidence in Mexican caves to suggest that humankind has been eating squash for at least 7,000 years.

• Butternut squash is a variety of winter squash. Other varieties include acorn, spaghetti and sweet squash.

• Winter squash develops more beta-carotene after being stored than it contains immediately after picking.

• The smallest butternut squashes are usually the tastiest.

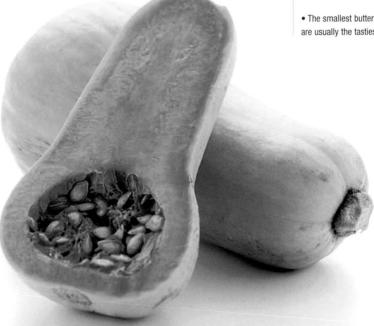

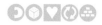

Sweet Potato

PROPERTIES/ACTIONS

- Boosts immunity
- Anti-cancer
- Complex carbohydrate
- Rich in fibre

PARTS USED

- Whole vegetable

Discovered by Columbus in the West Indies, orange-fleshed sweet potatoes are packed full of beta-carotene and other nutrients.

Sweet potatoes are rich in both beta-carotene and vitamin C, which boost immunity and help to prevent cardiovascular disease. These two powerful antioxidants also stave off some age-related conditions, particularly those of the eyes.

Beta-carotene can reduce the risk of cancer, especially endometrial cancer, while for those with respiratory problems, vitamin C acts on the lining of the lungs and makes breathing easier. Sweet potatoes are a complex carbohydrate and are rich in fibre, and can thus help to maintain blood-sugar levels.

SWEET POTATO CAKES

200g (7oz) sweet potato, cooked, with skin removed
100g (3½oz/1 cup) buckwheat flour
100g (3½oz/7 tbsp) margarine
1 apple, grated
1 tsp chopped ginger

Preheat the oven to 200°C/ 400°F/Gas 6. Combine all the ingredients well, then form into 4–8 balls. Arrange the balls on a greased baking sheet and flatten slightly. Bake for 30 minutes. Eat warm.

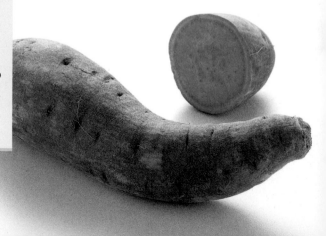

Potato

PROPERTIES/ACTIONS
- Anti-cancer
- High in fibre

PARTS USED
- Whole vegetable

Simple yet versatile, the potato is the world's number one vegetable crop and has long been used as a folk remedy.

Potatoes are a good source of complex carbohydrates, which help maintain blood sugar levels and boost energy. They are also high in vitamin C, which boosts immunity, and due to their potassium content they can help to control high blood pressure. Being rich in fibre they offer additional digestive benefits. The outer peel of potatoes contains chlorogenic acid, which acts as an anti-carcinogenic compound.

Its kinship with the deadly nightshade family made the potato feared when first discovered.

POTATO JUICE
for healthy digestion

250g (9oz) potatoes
lemon juice, to taste

Peel and scrub the potatoes, then chop into bite-sized pieces before liquidizing. Add lemon juice to taste. Take 2 tbsp before each meal. Do not take the juice for longer than 24 hours.

059

Onion

PROPERTIES/ACTIONS
- Protective
- Expectorant
- Anti-cancer
- Antibiotic

PARTS USED
- Whole vegetable, peeled

In medieval Europe bunches of onions were hung on doors to help ward off the plague.

A member of the allium family, onions have long played a central role in folk medicine and have a wealth of health-giving properties.

Onions are known to protect the circulatory system – they contain many compounds that help lower cholesterol, thin the blood and prevent the hardening of arteries. Rich in quercetin, onions may halt the progression of cancerous tumours and eliminate harmful bacteria in the gut. They also contain sulphur compounds that inhibit the inflammatory response, thus treating everything from insect bites to asthma.

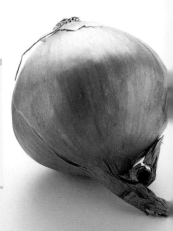

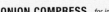

ONION COMPRESS *for inflamed wounds, headaches & earaches*

4 medium onions, peeled and finely chopped
white muslin or linen bag

Lightly steam the onions and wrap in the white muslin or linen bag. Apply to the inflamed area or aching parts. Once the compress cools down, replace it with another. Repeat up to four times in succession, or until the symptoms alleviate.

Okra

Okra can help the digestive system to recover from an upset stomach.

This vegetable, which looks like a mini green banana, is a staple in Middle Eastern cooking and regularly features in Indian, North African and Caribbean cuisine. Okra is a good source of soluble fibre, which helps to reduce cholesterol and stabilize blood sugar levels. It also contains psyllium, which acts as a probiotic in the gut, encouraging the growth of friendly bacteria and helping to soothe stomach upsets.

NUTRIENTS

Vitamins B1, B3, B5, B6, C, K, beta-carotene, folic acid (folate); calcium, iodine, iron, magnesium, manganese, phosphorus, potassium, selenium, zinc

---

VEGETABLE GUMBO

400g (14oz) okra, stems removed
2 courgettes (zucchini)
2 yellow (bell) peppers, deseeded
3 beef tomatoes
1 onion, finely chopped
1 tbsp sunflower oil
1 tbsp tomato purée (paste)
brown rice, to serve

Chop the vegetables into 2.5cm (1in) cubes. In an oven-proof dish, fry the onion, then the vegetables, in the oil until soft. Mix in the purée, cover and bake in a pre-heated oven at 190°C/375°F/Gas 5 for 1 hour. Serve with brown rice.

Because of their shape, okra are commonly known as ladies' fingers.

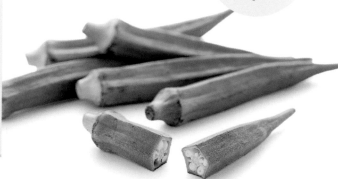

♥🍴🔄

Yam

A fabulous form of slow-releasing energy, this starchy root vegetable is a popular alternative to the potato in many parts of the world.

NUTRIENTS
Vitamins B1, B3, B5, B6, C, E, folic acid (folate); calcium, iodine, iron, magnesium, manganese, phosphorus, potassium, selenium, zinc

Thanks to their rich fibre content, yams rank lower on the glycaemic index and provide a more sustained form of carbohydrate energy than the more popular potatoes.

YAM FACTS

• One of the most widely consumed foods in the world, yams have been cultivated since 8000BCE in Africa and Asia.

• Yams come in yellow, white, ivory and purple varieties.

• There are more than 200 species of yam.

• Yams sometimes have offshoots, known as "toes".

• Unlike sweet potatoes, yams are toxic if eaten raw, although both are perfectly safe to eat when cooked.

BOOSTS ENERGY

High in potassium and low in sodium, yams help to regulate the fluid balance that exercise can so easily deplete through perspiration. Yam contains several of the B-vitamins and is particularly rich in vitamin B1, useful for boosting energy levels,

CITRUS YAMS

2 yams, peeled and chopped into 2.5cm (1in) chunks
4 tbsp olive oil
1 tbsp chopped parsley
1 tbsp chopped coriander (cilantro)
juice and zest of 1 orange
juice and zest of 1 lime

Steam the yam for 20 minutes until tender. In a bowl, whisk together the oil, parsley, coriander, and the juice and zest of the orange and lime. Fold the cooked yam into the dressing. Serve as a starter, a side-dish or a snack.

and manganese, a trace mineral that helps the body with the metabolism of carbohydrates.

BALANCES BLOOD SUGAR AND SALT

Discoretine, another chemical found in yam, is particularly useful as it reduces blood sugar and increases blood flow through the kidneys. This promotes the excretion of excess salt, which in turn helps to reduce high blood pressure.

YAM DUMPLINGS ROLLED IN POPPY SEEDS

1 yam, peeled and chopped
3 egg yolks
½ tsp chilli powder
1 tsp cornflour (cornstarch)
3 tbsp self-raising flour
4 tbsp poppy seeds

Boil the yam for 20 minutes until tender. Drain, allow to cool, then purée in a food processor. Transfer to a bowl and mix in the egg yolks, chilli and flours. Form into balls and roll in the poppy seeds. Line a steamer with foil, place over a pan of simmering water. Steam for 10 minutes and serve.

Never try to eat the skin of a yam, as it is woody and inedible.

Cauliflower

PROPERTIES/ACTIONS
- Anti-cancer
- Boosts immunity

PARTS USED
- Vegetable head

MEDITERRANEAN-STYLE CAULIFLOWER

1 medium cauliflower, separated into florets
5 black olives, pitted and finely chopped
1 tbsp chopped parsley
1 tsp red wine vinegar
pinch of crushed red pepper flakes

Put the cauliflower florets in a saucepan with 60ml (2fl oz/ ¼ cup) water. Cover and bring to the boil. Cook for 4–5 minutes, or until the cauliflower starts to soften. Stir in the olives, parsley, vinegar and pepper flakes. Cook for 1 minute or until heated through.

Like other members of the cabbage *(Cruciferae)* family, cauliflower is loaded with nutrients that seem to wage war against a host of diseases.

Cauliflower is a rich source of phytonutrients, thought to help stave off cancer. Sulforaphane steps up the production of enzymes that sweep toxins out of the body, while Indole-3-carbinol reduces levels of harmful oestrogens that can foster tumour growth, particularly in the breast and prostate gland.

Cauliflower is also packed with vitamin C and folic acid (folate), which are known for keeping the immune system strong.

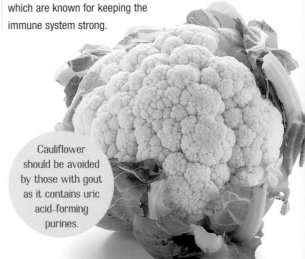

Cauliflower should be avoided by those with gout as it contains uric acid-forming purines.

063

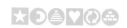

Rhubarb

Used in Chinese medicine for thousands of years, this relative of dock is a powerful disease-fighter.

This sharp-tasting food contains anti-bacterial chemicals that help the body to fight off infections. It's a good source of immune-supporting vitamin C, and contains compounds which help to prevent cancer. Rhubarb is high in dietary fibre. This is helpful for lowering cholesterol and preventing heart disease, and acts as a natural laxative. It also contains oxalic acid, which is thought to aid the body to detoxify. Rhubarb should be avoided by those prone to gout and arthritis, as oxalates can worsen these conditions.

NUTRIENTS

Vitamin C, folic acid (folate); calcium, magnesium, potassium; fibre; oxalic acid

---

RHUBARB CRUMBLE

serves 4

5 stalks rhubarb, chopped
125g (4½oz/⅔ cup) raw cane sugar
175g (6oz/1½ cups) plain (all-purpose) flour
100g (3½oz/½ cup) unsalted butter

Preheat the oven to 180°C/350°F/Gas 4. Place the rhubarb, and half the sugar in a saucepan with 2 tbsp water and stew for 5 minutes. Meanwhile, make the topping – rub the butter into the flour until it forms the consistency of bread crumbs, then add the remaining sugar and stir. Pour the stewed rhubarb into an ovenproof dish, spoon the crumble on top and cook in the oven until golden.

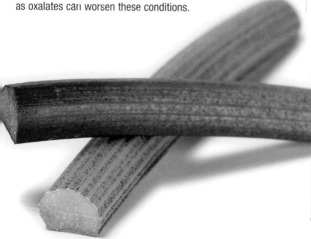

064

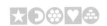

Shiitake

NUTRIENTS
Vitamins B1, B2, B3, C; iron, magnesium, phosphorous, potassium; lentinan; protein

These highly-prized Japanese tree fungi have powerful disease-fighting capabilities.

Native to China, Japan and Korea, shiitake mushrooms have been used in those countries for thousands of years to prevent and treat illness. In ancient China they were prescribed by physicians to help beat a range of conditions, from colds and 'flu to gastrointestinal problems. Recently, shiitake mushrooms have been the subject of several scientific studies that are researching their pro-immunity and healing powers.

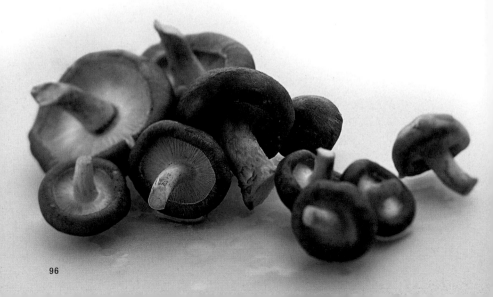

SHIITAKE'S IMMUNITY-BOOSTING PROPERTIES

These fungi contain lentinan, a polysaccharide compound that has been shown to help lower cholesterol. Lentinan has also been isolated and licensed as an anti-cancer drug in Japan because of its ability to stimulate the immune system to deactivate malignant cells. In addition lentinan is understood to trigger the production of the anti-viral and anti-bacterial substance interferon, which may help to inhibit the progress of the virus HIV. The mushrooms are also rich in the amino acids that enhance general immune function.

USING SHIITAKE MUSHROOM

Shiitake mushrooms are more expensive than many varieties, but a small amount gives health benefits and satisfies appetite. They can be bought fresh, pickled or dried, and can be used in dishes in the same way as ordinary field mushrooms.

SHIITAKE FACTS

• In ancient China, shiitake mushrooms were prized so highly that they were reserved for consumption by the emperor and his family.

• Shiitake is one of a number of medicinal mushrooms which, more than any other food, are currently being studied for their pro-immunity properties. Other well researched fungi are maitake and reishi.

• The health-boosting benefits of shiitake are now available in supplement form but as they have anti-bloodclotting properties those on blood thinning medication should avoid excessive amounts.

SHIITAKE NOODLES *serves 4*

250g (9oz) thick egg noodles
3 tbsp soy sauce
1 tbsp oyster sauce
1 tsp brown sugar
1 tbsp sesame oil
2 small red chillies, sliced and deseeded
1 packet firm tofu, diced
2 garlic cloves, crushed

5cm (2in) piece fresh ginger, grated
150g (5½oz) fresh shiitake mushrooms, sliced
6 spring onions (scallions), chopped

Cover the noodles in boiling water and leave to soften for 5 minutes.

Drain. In a bowl, mix together the soy sauce, oyster sauce and sugar. Heat the oil in a wok. Stir-fry the chillies, tofu, garlic and ginger for 2 minutes, then add the noodles, mushrooms, sauce mixture and spring onions. Toss together and serve immediately.

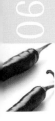

✚ ❤ ◐ ✦

Chilli

PROPERTIES/ACTIONS
- Stimulant
- Carminative
- Antiseptic
- Expectorant
- Decongestant
- Analgesic

PARTS USED
- Fresh & dried chilli

CHILLI PASTE
for colds & bronchial conditions

3 small Thai dried chillies
2 garlic cloves, halved
1 small onion, chopped
30g (1oz/2½ tbsp) sugar
50ml (1¾fl oz/3½ tbsp) lemon
juice
½ tsp salt

Put all the ingredients in a blender with 50ml (1¾fl oz/3½ tbsp) water and whizz until finely chopped. Pour the mixture into a small pan and cook gently, stirring occasionally, for 10 minutes.

According to traditional Oriental theory, "If you have a cold, you can build a fire in your stomach" with a spice such as chilli.

Chilli is a hot, pungent yang spice and a highly effective decongestant for colds as well as respiratory disorders. It flushes out the sinuses and clears the lungs, thus treating various bronchial conditions.

Chilli also acts on the circulatory and digestive systems, and is used to treat a wide range of complaints ranging from arthritis and chilblains to colic and diarrhoea.

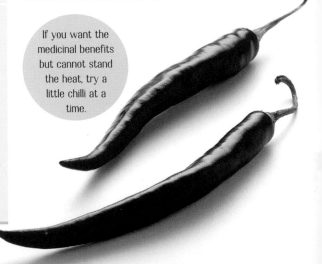

If you want the medicinal benefits but cannot stand the heat, try a little chilli at a time.

Seaweed

Seaweed is a marine algae, the oldest form of life on the planet, and it contains a host of health-giving properties, particularly minerals.

Seaweed is rich in minerals such as potassium, magnesium, calcium and iron, as well as trace elements, and benefits many body systems. Due to its high iodine content, it aids digestion and soothes ulcers. It also promotes the functioning of the thyroid and metabolism. Seaweed is filled with mucilaginous gels that alkalinize the blood, treating rheumatic complaints. It also helps clear liver stagnation, treating PMS, headaches and skin problems. Seaweed is an excellent lymphatic cleanser.

PROPERTIES/ACTIONS
- High in iodine
- Supports thyroid & metabolism
- Mucilaginous
- Clears liver stagnation
- Lymphatic cleanser

PARTS USED
- Whole plant

SEAWEED RICE

2 tbsp wakame
½ medium onion, chopped
2 large garlic cloves, minced
200g (7oz/1 cup) brown rice

Rinse the wakame, and soak in the 625ml (20fl oz/2½ cups) warm water for 5 minutes. Squeeze dry and chop. Save the water and heat 1 tbsp in a pan. Sauté the onion gently for 2 minutes, stirring. Add all the other ingredients and the remaining water. Bring to the boil, then simmer for 35 minutes. Serve.

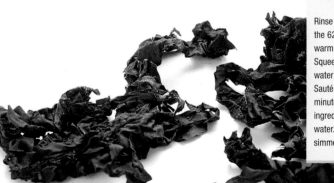

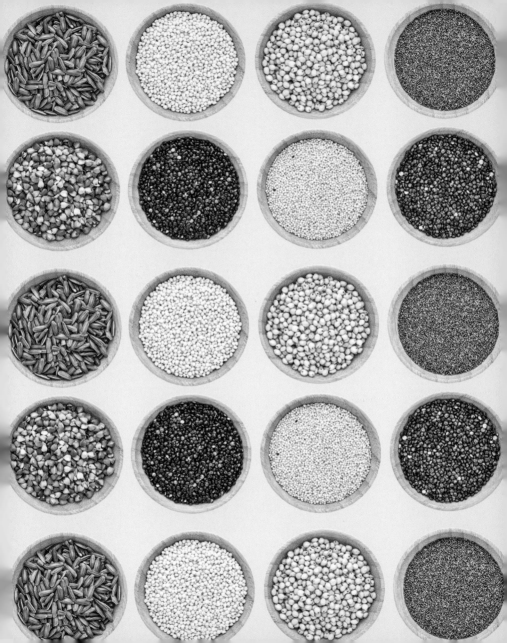

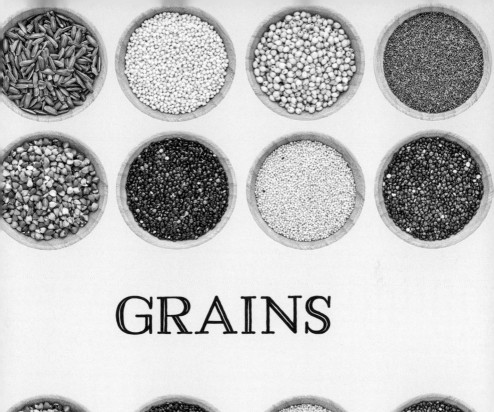

GRAINS

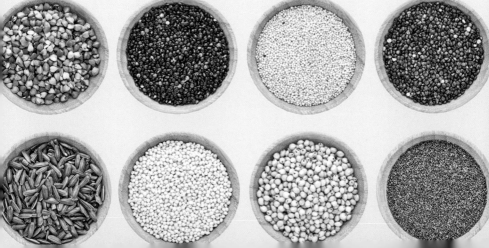

Rice

NUTRIENTS
Vitamins B1, B3, folic acid (folate); iron, magnesium, manganese, phosphorous, copper, zinc; complex carbohydrates, fibre, protein

The second most widely cultivated grain in the world is a powerhouse of nutrients.

Brown rice is dense in B-vitamins, which are needed for a healthy brain and nervous system, while its protein levels help to build muscles, skin and hair. It is also a good source of zinc and trace minerals, such as magnesium, phosphorus and copper, which all build resistance to infections. Rice's rich fibre content is excellent for the digestive system and helps to lower cholesterol, so is important for a healthy heart. It is a complex carbohydrate, so it releases energy slowly, and is ideal for keeping hunger pangs at bay.

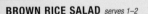

BROWN RICE SALAD *serves 1–2*

55g (2oz/⅓ cup) brown rice, cooked and cooled
2 spring onions (scallions), sliced
4 tomatoes, cut into segments
100g (3½oz/1 cup) black olives, pitted and halved
3 tbsp chopped basil

2 garlic cloves, crushed
3 tbsp olive oil

Combine all the ingredients together in a large salad bowl. Leave, unrefrigerated, for 1 hour to allow the flavours to mingle, then serve.

Wild Rice

Chewy in texture, wild rice is rich in protein, packed with dietary fibre and low in fat.

Wild rice is not really rice, but a type of grass containing twice the protein of white rice and fewer calories and fat. Nutritionally, it is one of the few grains that also provide the essential fatty acids omega-3 and -6, which are mostly found in oily fish, nuts and seeds. It's also an excellent source of the energy-boosting B-vitamins, thiamine (B1), riboflavin (B2) and niacin (B3).

NUTRIENTS
Vitamins B1, B2, B3, E; iodine, phosphorus, potassium, selenium, zinc; omega-3 and -6 essential fatty acids

Always choose brown or wild rice, which is richer in nutrients than the processed, white variety.

SALMON AND WILD RICE STEW

2 red onions, finely chopped
1 tbsp olive oil
100g (3½oz/½ cup) wild rice
750ml (26fl oz/3 cups) fish stock
100g (3½oz/½ cup) basmati rice
500g (1lb 2oz) salmon fillets, cut into large pieces
handful of dill, chopped
2 tbsp crème fraîche

In a pan, fry the onions in the oil until soft. Stir in the wild rice and stock. Bring to the boil and cook for 15 minutes. Add the basmati rice, cover, reduce the heat and cook for 20 minutes. Add the salmon. Cook for 7 minutes. Flake the salmon, then add the dill and crème fraîche.

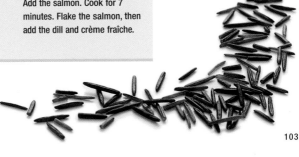

Rye

Grown in Russia for more than 2,000 years, rye is commonly milled into flour and is used as a nutritious alternative to wheat.

PROPERTIES/ACTIONS
- Rich in calcium & iron
- Highly digestible
- Prebiotic qualities

PARTS USED
- Whole grain

High in calcium, iron and potassium, the rye grain is good for osteoporosis, anaemia and headaches. It is also rich in plant lignans, which help to reduce blood viscosity. Containing dietary fibre, rye may relieve constipation. Rye also contains sucrose and fructooligosaccharide, which have prebiotic properties that are useful to digestive health.

RYE PANCAKES

100g (3½oz/⅔ cup) rye flour
1 large egg
150ml (5fl oz/⅔ cup) milk
1 tbsp olive oil

Whizz the rye flour, egg, milk and 100ml (3½fl oz/scant ½ cup) water in a food processor. Leave to stand for 10–15 minutes. Drizzle some oil into a heavy frying pan and heat. Carefully ladle in the batter, allowing 2–3 tbsp per pancake. As the mixture for each pancake begins to bubble on the surface, flip it over and leave for 4–5 minutes, or until cooked through.

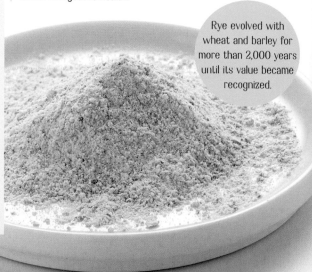

Rye evolved with wheat and barley for more than 2,000 years until its value became recognized.

070

Bulgur Wheat

NUTRIENTS
Vitamins B1, B2, B3; copper, iron, magnesium, phosphorous; protein, fibre

A mineral-rich grain made from wheat berries, bulgur makes a good alternative to rice.

A cracked wheat grain, bulgur is dense in digestion-boosting fibre, which is also needed to keep blood cholesterol low. It is a good source of B-vitamins, which help the body to mop up invader cells, as well as stabilising energy levels and maintaining a healthy nervous system. Bulgur wheat also contains minerals including iron, important for increasing overall resistance to infection.

BULGUR-STUFFED VINE LEAVES serves 4

100ml (3½fl oz/scant ½ cup) boiling water
150g (5½oz/¾ cup) bulgur wheat
1 small onion, sliced
3 tsp olive oil
1 tsp cumin seeds
55g (2oz) tofu, grated
6 sun-dried tomatoes, chopped
1 tsp chopped mint
½ tsp lemon juice
black pepper
16 vine leaves, blanched for 5 minutes

Pour the water onto the bulgur wheat, and set aside for 20 minutes. Fry the onion in the oil until golden, then stir in the cumin seeds. Remove from the heat and add the bulgur wheat, tofu, tomatoes, mint, lemon juice and pepper. Divide the mixture among the vine leaves, roll and secure with a cocktail stick. Steam for 20 minutes and serve.

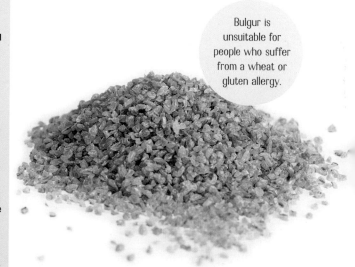

Bulgur is unsuitable for people who suffer from a wheat or gluten allergy.

071

Quinoa

Pronounced "keen-waa", quinoa is one of the best sources of protein in the plant kingdom.

Strictly speaking, quinoa is a seed, not a grain. Low in fat, it's full of slow-release carbohydrates, which balance the blood sugar.

BUILDS STRENGTH

Containing all eight essential amino acids, quinoa is an exceptionally rich source of protein, making it a useful addition to the diet of regular exercisers and serious athletes, who need more protein

NUTRIENTS
Vitamins B1, B2, B3, B5, B6, E, folic acid (folate); calcium, copper, iron, magnesium, manganese, phosphorus, potassium, zinc

QUINOA FACTS
• Quinoa was once called "the gold of the Incas", who recognized its value in increasing the stamina of their warriors.

• When quinoa is cooked, the grains become translucent and the white germ partially detaches itself, appearing like a white-spiralled tail.

• For a nuttier flavour, dry roast quinoa before cooking in a heavy-based pan over a medium-low heat, stirring constantly for 5 minutes.

• The leaves of the quinoa plant are edible, with a taste similar to its green-leafed relatives, spinach and chard.

QUINOA-STUFFED PEPPERS

250g (9oz/½ cup) quinoa
1 onion, chopped
2 garlic cloves, crushed
115g (4oz) mushrooms, chopped into small pieces
1 tbsp olive oil
4 red (bell) peppers

In a pan, bring 500ml (17fl oz/ 2 cups) water to the boil. Add the quinoa, reduce the heat and simmer for 15 minutes.

In another pan, soften the onion, garlic and mushrooms in the oil. Add the quinoa and mix well. Cut the tops off the peppers and remove the cores and seeds. Fill each pepper with the mixture, replace the tops and place in an ovenproof dish. Bake in a pre-heated oven at 190°C/375°F/Gas 5 for 45 minutes.

than inactive people. (An insufficient intake delays the body's recovery after training and slows the development of muscle and stamina.)

BOOSTS ENERGY

A serving of quinoa provides nearly the entire spectrum of B-vitamins, needed to boost energy and combat stress, as well as lots of vitamin E, a key component in skin health and the body's healing process. Quinoa is also rich in calcium and magnesium, essential for healthy bones, iron to help prevent fatigue, and zinc to enhance the immune system.

Quinoa is loaded with lysine, an amino acid that is essential for tissue growth and repair.

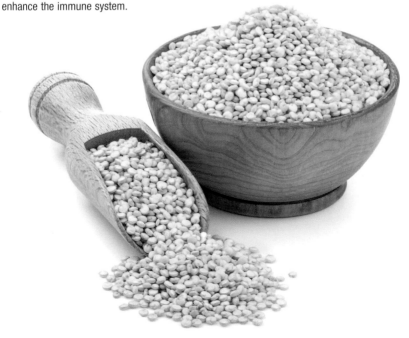

072

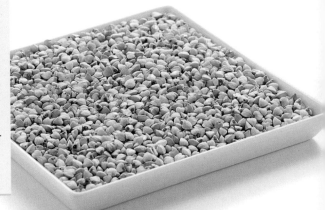

Buckwheat

A staple in Russia and Poland, buckwheat, although commonly considered a grain, is, in fact, a nut with unique health-giving abilities.

Buckwheat is high in the bioflavonoid rutin, which strengthens blood capillaries and is an especially good food for the prevention and treatment of varicose veins, frostbite and chilblains. Rutin may be particularly important in the treatment of high blood pressure and hardening of the arteries, and it is also thought to lift depression.

Applied topically, buckwheat helps to draw out excess fluid from the tissues, thus helping to relieve pain and inflammation.

PROPERTIES/ACTIONS
- Strengthens blood capillaries
- Prevents varicose veins
- Draws out excess fluid

PARTS USED
- Whole grain

BUCKWHEAT POULTICE
for skin inflammation

220g (7½oz/1⅓ cup) buckwheat flour

Boil 250ml (9fl oz/1 cup) water in a saucepan. Allow to cool a little, then add the flour and mix well to form a paste. Wrap the paste in a piece of muslin (cheesecloth). Apply directly to the affected area and hold in place with a bandage. Leave for 10 minutes, or until the paste begins to cool, then reheat and apply for another 10 minutes.

Barley

A staple in the Middle Ages, barley is valued as a traditional remedy for its demulcent qualities and ability to cleanse the lymphatic system.

Barley has a unique ability to act on the mucous membranes, and may therefore help to soothe inflammatory conditions of the intestines and the urinary tract. Barley is rich in minerals, with high levels of calcium and potassium and plenty of B-complex vitamins, and it is useful for people suffering from stress or fatigue. It also contains beta-glucan, a gummy fibre that has dramatic cholesterol-lowering abilities.

Dioscorides said that barley could "weaken and restrain all sore and ulcerated throats".

PROPERTIES/ACTIONS
- Demulcent
- Cleansing
- Anti-stress

PARTS USED
- Whole grain

LEMON BARLEY WATER
for cystitis, constipation & diarrhoea

**125g (4oz/⅝ cup) pearl barley
grated zest of 1 lemon
honey, to taste**

Bring the pearl barley to a boil in a saucepan with 240ml (8fl oz/1 cup) of water. Strain, then add another 660ml (22fl oz/2¾ cups) water and the lemon zest. Simmer until the barley is soft, adding more water as required. Strain the liquid, sweeten with honey and leave to cool. Drink the lemon barley water when symptoms arise.

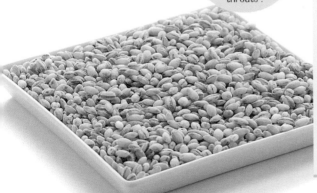

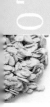

Oats

PROPERTIES/ACTIONS
- Nerve tonic
- Eases digestive problems
- Anti-depressant
- Prevents heart disease
- Anti-spasmodic
- Emollient

PARTS USED
- Whole grain

OATEN JELLY
for gastric problems

65g (2½oz/½ cup) oat flour
15g (½oz/1 tbsp) butter
sugar or honey, to taste

Blend the oat flour with 50ml (1¾fl oz/3½ tbsp) water. Boil another 400ml (14fl oz/1¾ cups) water in a pan and slowly pour onto the flour, stirring until thick. Return the mixture to the pan and add the butter. Bring to the boil and simmer for 7 minutes, stirring continuously, until thick. Add sugar or honey.

Oats are highly nutritious and are a traditional remedy for soothing nervous conditions and aiding digestive complaints.

Although their native country is unknown, oats are said to be indigenous to Sicily and Chile. The grain is commonly "rolled" to be used as a commercial foodstuff, and when the seed is kiln dried, stripped of its husk and delicate outer skin, and then coarsely ground, it constitutes the oatmeal of Scotland.

Oats provide a cornucopia of nourishment – they are a good source of protein, and are incredibly high in calcium, potassium and magnesium which, like the B vitamins, act as a nerve tonic, as well as promoting strong bones and teeth. They are also rich in fibre and singularly digestible, as well as having a demulcent quality that protects the duodenal surfaces, stomach and intestines. Oats are especially good for irritable bowel syndrome since they are anti-spasmodic.

Oats have plenty of silicon for maintaining healthy arterial walls, and beta-glucan, a soluble fibre that overcomes high blood pressure. Oat bran, meanwhile, has become well known for combating high levels of blood cholesterol.

Oats are a complex carbohydrate with a very low glycaemic index (GI). They therefore provide sustainable energy, alleviating insomnia and improving insulin sensitivity in people with diabetes.

They also have a mild tranquillizing effect, and are a reliable remedy for depression.

When applied locally, oats have an emollient effect, and when combined with water in the bath, they can help to alleviate skin irritations.

In 1652 Nicholas Culpeper said, "A poultice made of meal of oats and some oil of bay, helpeth the itch."

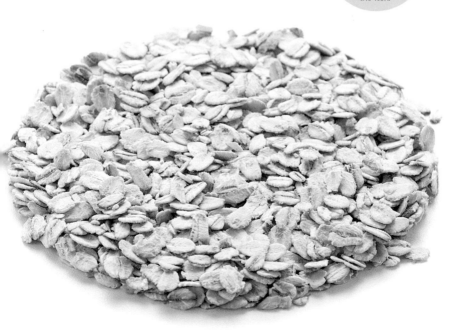

Wheatgerm

NUTRIENTS
Vitamins B1, B2, B3, B5, B6, E, folic acid (folate); iron, magnesium, manganese, selenium, zinc, fibre

You should avoid wheatgerm if you are allergic to wheat or gluten.

This tiny wheat seed is surprisingly rich in essential nutrients.

Found inside the wheat grain, wheatgerm is rich in the antioxidant vitamin E, which helps to detoxify the body by neutralising harmful free radicals. It is also an excellent source of a range of B-vitamins, which are needed by the body's cells to fight disease as well as to maintain healthy nerves and mucous membranes. Wheatgerm is a very high-fibre food, and so helps to ensure an efficient digestive system as well as reduce cholesterol levels.

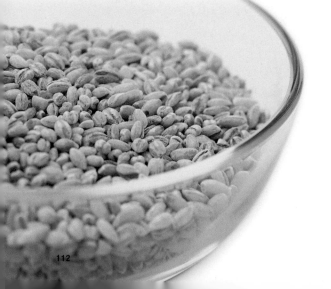

HONEY WHEATGERM SMOOTHIE

200ml (7fl oz/¾ cup) soya milk
55g (2oz/¼ cup) plain bio-yogurt
125g (4½oz) strawberries, hulled
1 large ripe banana
2 tsp wheatgerm
2 tsp manuka honey

Whizz all the ingredients in a blender and serve.

Millet

Millet is a highly nutritious grain that supplies fantastic support to the digestive system, especially the stomach, spleen and pancreas.

PROPERTIES/ACTIONS
- Carminative
- Counteracts acidity
- Contains silicon

PARTS USED
- Whole grain

High in protein and low in starch, millet supports the digestive system as it is the only alkaline grain. It has anti-fungal and anti-mucus properties, which help to prevent ailments such as candida and premenstrual discomfort. Millet is rich in silicon, the great cleansing, mending and eliminating mineral salt, essential for hair, skin, teeth, eye and nail health. Silicon also supports arterial health. It has high levels of potassium and magnesium, useful for treating arthritis and osteoporosis.

SEASONAL VEGETABLE & MILLET STEW

375g (13oz/1½ cups) millet
1kg (2lb 4oz) seasonal
  vegetables of your choice,
  chopped into bite-size pieces
vegetable oil, for frying
2 litres (70fl oz/8 cups) boiling
  water
2 tsp vegetable bouillon powder

Place the vegetables in a large pan with a little oil and sauté until soft. Roast the millet separately in a little oil for 3–4 minutes, until brown. Add to the vegetables and sauté a little longer, stirring. Add the water and bouillon powder. Simmer for about 30 minutes. Add extra seasoning if desired. Serve hot.

Triticale

NUTRIENTS
Vitamins B1, folic acid (folate);
calcium, iron, magnesium

A nutritious alternative to wheat, triticale is a great source of carbohydrate, boosting stamina.

Triticale is a hybrid of wheat and rye that was first bred in Sweden and Scotland in the late nineteenth century. Today, cracked triticale can be used in the same way as cracked wheat, and triticale flakes make a great substitute for oat flakes. It is high in folic acid (folate), which protects against heart disease, as well as calcium and magnesium, crucial for healthy bones.

The word "triticale" is an amalgamation of the Latin words triticum (wheat) and secale (rye).

MUSHROOM BAKE

1 onion, finely chopped
500g (1lb 2oz) mushrooms,
   halved
1 tbsp olive oil
100g (3½oz/heaped ¾ cup)
   triticale flour
1 tbsp tomato purée (paste)
handful of oregano

In a pan, fry the onion and mushrooms in the oil. In a bowl, mix the flour and tomato purée with 4 tbsp water to form a paste. Add the oregano and mix all the ingredients together. Transfer to an oven-proof dish and bake in a pre-heated oven at 170°C/325°F/Gas 3 for 20 minutes.

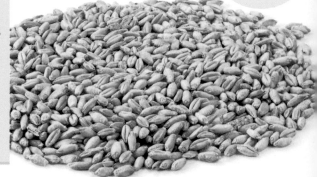

Wild Oats

Nutrient-rich wild oats will boost your energy and help combat the effects of stress.

Rich in protein, calcium, magnesium, silica and iron, and a host of vitamins, oats help to make bones and teeth strong. Both strengthening and relaxing, oats can help to relieve depression, anxiety, tension, insomnia and nervous exhaustion. They also lower blood cholesterol and sugar, helping to prevent heart problems and diabetes. High in fibre, oats are great for combating constipation, and by removing toxins from the bowel are said to help prevent bowel cancer. Use oatmeal externally to soothe inflamed skin conditions.

PARTS USED
- Grains

PROPERTIES/ACTIONS
- Nervine
- Nourishing tonic
- Antidepressant
- Hypoglycemic
- Demulcent
- Vulnerary
- Hormone-regulating
- Cholesterol-lowering

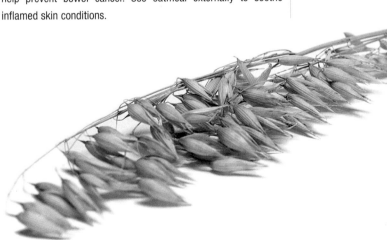

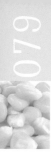

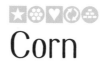

Corn

NUTRIENTS
Vitamins A, B3, B5, C, beta-carotene, folic acid (folate); magnesium, zinc; fibre

Also known as maize, this staple food is particularly rich in immunity-bolstering vitamins.

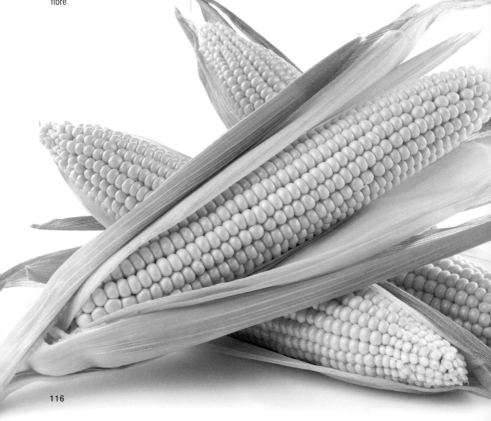

Corn can be ground into cornflour (cornstarch) and used for its thickening properties in cooking, particularly in sauces and stews. It is most nutritious in its unprocessed form, as sweetcorn – the bright yellow cobs that are surrounded with lusciously sweet kernels. Sweetcorn contains good levels of vitamin C, which helps to strengthen the immune system to fight viruses and bacteria, and is an overall excellent source of fibre, which is important for lowering blood cholesterol and helping with the prevention of heart disease. Folic acid (folate), needed for reproductive health, is found in corn, along with other B-vitamins that are useful for boosting energy and resistance to stress.

Canned and frozen sweetcorn retains most of the nutrients found in the fresh cobs.

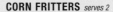

CORN FRITTERS *serves 2*

115g (4oz/¾ cup) wholemeal flour
2 eggs
300ml (10½fl oz/1¼ cups) milk
2 tbsp chopped coriander (cilantro)
225g (8oz) sweetcorn, fresh or canned
black pepper
2 tbsp olive oil

Whisk the flour, eggs and milk into a smooth batter, then add the coriander, sweetcorn and pepper. Heat the olive oil in a frying pan, divide the mixture into 8 small patties, and fry until golden on both sides. Serve.

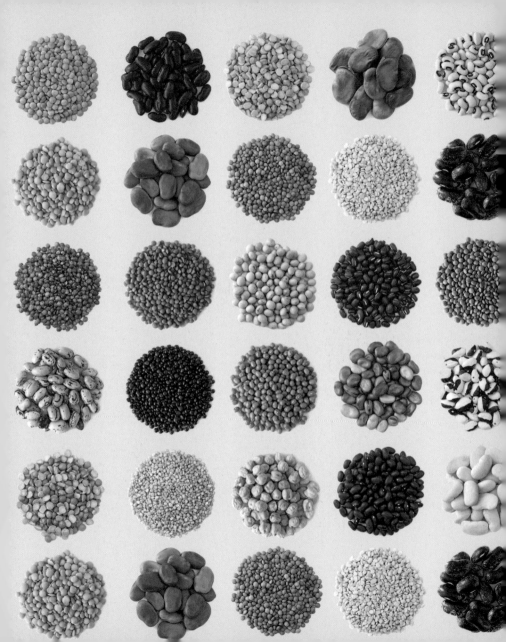

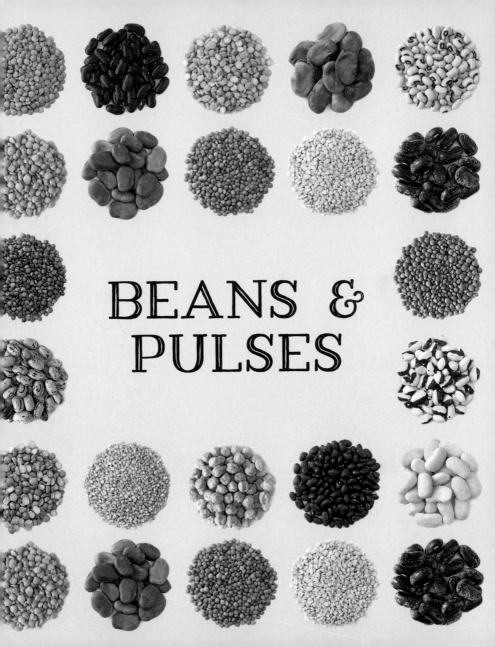

BEANS & PULSES

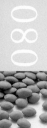

NATURE'S PHARMACY

Lentil

A staple food in many countries, lentils have a rich history of use and are one of the single best-known, nutritious and digestible foods.

PROPERTIES/ACTIONS
- High in protein
- Regulates nervous system
- Rich in fibre

PARTS USED
- Whole lentil

Whether red, green or brown, lentils are a good source of protein. They contain high levels of B vitamins, particularly B3, deficiency of which can lead to poor memory and irritability. They are also rich in iron and are recommended for pregnant and lactating women, as well as those suffering from anaemia.

Lentils are a good source of fibre and help to regulate colon function, as well as the circulatory system.

SPICY LENTIL BURGERS

175g (6oz/⅞ cup) red lentils
1 tbsp olive oil
1 onion, finely chopped
1–2 tsp curry powder
450ml (16fl oz/2 cups)
  vegetable stock
125g (4oz/1 cup) wholemeal
  breadcrumbs

Fry the onion in the oil, then stir in the curry powder and cook for 2 minutes. Add the lentils and stock. Bring to the boil, then simmer for 20–25 minutes. Add the breadcrumbs and shape into four burgers. Grill (broil) on a lightly oiled baking tray until crisp and brown.

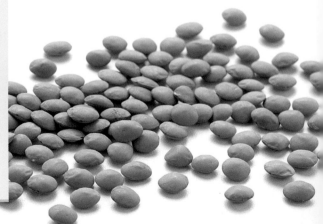

Sprouts

PROPERTIES/ACTIONS
- Rich in enzymes
- Dense in nutrients
- Highly digestible
- Anti-cancer

PARTS USED
- Whole sprout

SPROUT SALAD

200g (7oz/2 cups) mung bean
    sprouts
200g (7oz/2 cups) alfalfa
    sprouts
50g (2oz/¼ cup) fenugreek
    sprouts
1 medium lettuce, finely
    chopped
50g (2oz/¼ cup) finely chopped
    sunflower greens (baby
    plants from unhulled seeds
    grown in soil)
favourite salad dressing,
    to taste

Put all the salad vegetables in
a bowl. Season with the salad
dressing. Toss and serve.

First discovered by Chinese physicians more than 5,000 years ago, sprouts are full of all kinds of health-promoting enzymes, nutrients and sugars.

As a seed, sprouts' powerful enzymes that otherwise lie dormant are released. The starches within seeds are also converted into natural sugars. Sprouts are easily digested and assimilated, and provide more nutrients gram for gram than any other natural food known. They help every cell in the body to function efficiently. Because sprouts are generally high in vitamin C, they are useful in boosting immunity. Some sprouts are believed to have anti-cancer properties.

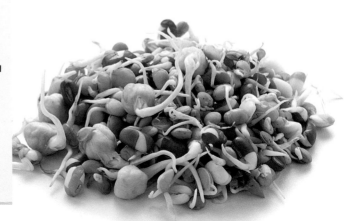

Soya Bean

PROPERTIES/ACTIONS
- Rich in protein
- Lowers cholesterol
- Source of phyto-oestrogens
- Low GI
- Combats stress

PARTS USED
- Whole bean

Originating in Japan, soya beans are made into a number of food products with a wealth of ancient medicinal properties.

Soya beans can be included in the diet in the form of soya oil, soya flour, tofu, tempeh, soya milk, textured vegetable protein (TVP), miso and soya sauce, and are often used instead of meat or dairy protein. Being rich in lecithin, a natural emulsifier of fats, they can assist in lowering cholesterol levels. Plant-derived protein is also said to help guard against gallstones.

Perhaps best known for their phyto-oestrogen content, soya beans are said to reduce symptoms of menopause and osteoporosis. They are excellent in promoting healthy colon and bowel function, and are protective against constipation, diverticular disease and haemorrhoids.

SOYA BEAN PÂTÉ

200g (7oz/1 cup) cooked soya
  beans
1 tbsp olive oil
1 medium onion, finely chopped
2 tbsp tomato purée (paste)
10 black olives, pitted and
  chopped

2 tbsp chopped parsley
1 tbsp sesame seeds, lightly
  toasted
pinch of salt

Put the soya beans in a bowl
and mash them with a fork. Heat

the olive oil in a frying pan and
sauté the onion until it is clear
and soft. Add to the beans.
Stir in the tomato purée, olives,
parsley, sesame seeds and salt.
Chill for at least 30 minutes
before serving.

Soya beans have a low glycaemic index (GI) and are great blood sugar and insulin regulators, which makes them useful in maintaining energy levels and for diabetics. They are also a valuable source of B-complex vitamins, which support the nervous system and help to combat stress.

SOYA PANCAKES

125g (4½oz/1 cup) soya flour
345g (12oz/2¾ cups) plain
  (all-purpose) flour
3 tbsp baking powder
3 tbsp sugar
½ tsp salt
3 eggs
750ml (24fl oz/3 cups) soya
  milk
6 tbsp soya oil
knob of butter

Combine all the ingredients, except the butter, in a bowl and beat to form a batter. Melt the butter in a frying pan and add ½ cup of batter. Cook on both sides until golden brown. Fold and serve.

Aduki bean

NUTRIENTS
Vitamins B1, B2, B3; calcium, magnesium, manganese, zinc; fibre, protein

ADUKI BEAN CASSEROLE
serves 2

1 red onion, chopped
2 tbsp olive oil
1 red (bell) pepper, chopped
1 stick celery, chopped
2 carrots, chopped
2 large tomatoes, chopped
200g (7oz) aduki beans, soaked overnight
1 garlic clove, crushed
1 tsp ground cumin
1 tsp fennel seeds
1 tsp ground coriander
600ml (21fl oz/2½ cups) vegetable bouillon

In a wok, gently stir-fry the onion in the olive oil until soft and golden. Add the pepper, celery, carrots and tomato, and stir-fry for 2 minutes. Add the beans, garlic and spices. Stir, pour on the bouillon and simmer for 30 minutes. Serve with brown rice.

These nutty beans, known as the "king of beans" in Japan, are packed with energising nutrients.

Aduki beans are high in fibre, making them useful for speeding up the elimination of waste and helping to detoxify the body. They contain good levels of B-vitamins, which are needed for steady energy production and to repair body tissues. Aduki beans are also a useful source of protein, which helps to build muscle and maintain healthy skin, and are rich in immunity minerals including anti-viral zinc, calcium and magnesium.

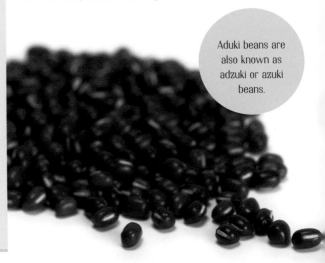

Aduki beans are also known as adzuki or azuki beans.

Black Bean

Originating in Peru, black beans are often used in the Creole and Cajun cuisines of North America and are highly nutritious.

Black beans are a source of complex carbohydrates, useful for many ailments, including heart problems. Rich in iron, they are known to help anaemia and to impart strength when recovering from illness. They are a rich source of energy-providing potassium, as well as folic acid (folate), which may lower the risk of heart disease and fight birth defects. They act on the reproductive organs and blood, and are useful for gynaecological problems.

PROPERTIES/ACTIONS
• Rich in iron
• Promotes reproductive health

PARTS USED
• Whole bean

BLACK BEAN DIP

300g (10½oz/1½ cups) black
   beans, cooked
1 small carrot, diced
1 small piece of celery, diced
1 tbsp minced garlic
1 tsp dried oregano
1 tsp ground cumin
½ tsp ground coriander
¼ tsp salt
125g (4½oz/½ cup) sour cream

Whizz all the ingredients in a blender. Transfer to a serving bowl. Cover and chill in the refrigerator until needed.

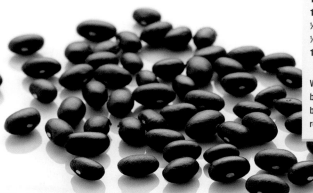

Black-eyed Bean

NUTRIENTS
Vitamins B1, B2, B3, biotin, folic acid (folate); calcium, iron, magnesium, manganese, selenium, zinc; fibre, protein

This highly nutritious bean is an essential ingredient in Creole and Cajun cooking.

Black-eyed beans contain zinc, an important antioxidant mineral that helps the development of the body's disease-fighting cells. They also contain selenium, another antioxidant mineral which is needed to produce antibodies and to help to prevent cancer. The beans are rich in energy-boosting B-vitamins, including folic acid (folate), which is necessary for healthy reproductive organs. They are also a good source of protein, used for building muscle and increasing vitality, and fibre, for a healthy digestive system and heart.

BLACK-EYED BEAN RICE *serves 4*

5 spring onions (scallions), chopped
2 tsp olive oil
350g (12oz) black-eyed beans, cooked
juice of 1 lime
½ tsp chilli powder
½ tsp cumin
2 tbsp chopped coriander (cilantro)
black pepper

150g (5½oz/¾ cup) basmati rice, cooked

Gently fry the onions in the oil until golden. Add the remaining ingredients, apart from the rice, along with 2 tbsp water, stir and heat through for 2 minutes. Add the rice and pepper and stir-fry for a further 2 minutes, then serve immediately.

Kidney Bean

Widely used in South America, these soft beans are high in protein, vitamins and minerals.

Kidney beans are rich in folic acid (folate), a B-vitamin that is important for good reproductive health and efficient wound healing. They are an excellent source of protein, which helps to keep energy levels steady, and contain high levels of fibre, which is vital for keeping blood cholesterol low, and good digestion. Kidney beans also contain iron – essential for the production of the immune system's antibodies and white blood cells.

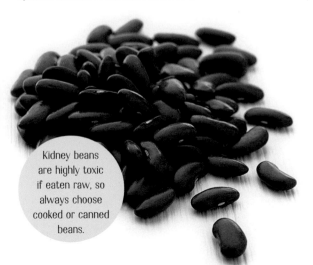

Kidney beans are highly toxic if eaten raw, so always choose cooked or canned beans.

NUTRIENTS

Folic acid (folate); potassium, iron, manganese; fibre, protein

QUICK KIDNEY BEAN CASSEROLE *serves 2*

2 tbsp olive oil
400g (14oz) canned kidney
    beans, drained
3 large ripe tomatoes, chopped
1 red (bell) pepper, chopped
1 onion, chopped
2 garlic cloves, crushed
1 courgette (zucchini), sliced
4 portabello mushrooms,
    sliced
2 tsp basil, chopped
1 tsp sea salt

Heat the olive oil in a large saucepan, then add the onion and stir-fry until golden. Add the pepper, courgette, mushrooms, tomato and garlic, stir for 5 minutes, then add the kidney beans, and enough water to cover. Add the basil and salt, then cover and simmer until the vegetables are soft. Serve with brown rice.

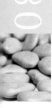

087

NATURE'S PHARMACY

Butterbean

This soft, floury bean is rich in B-vitamins and is a good source of protein.

Butterbeans have high levels of vitamin B5, an important immune stimulant that helps the body to produce antibodies to fight off disease. They are also a useful source of folic acid (folate), another B-vitamin that is vital for good reproductive health. In addition, butterbeans are rich in minerals, and have some manganese – which works to help stop viruses developing – as well as immune-fortifying iron and zinc.

Butterbeans are helpful for maintaining healthy skin and hair.

NUTRIENTS

Vitamins B3, B5, folic acid (folate); iron, manganese, potassium, zinc; fibre, protein

MIDDLE-EASTERN STYLE BEANS *serves 4*

1 onion, chopped
1 tsp ground cinnamon
2 tbsp olive oil
500g (1lb 2oz) cooked or canned butterbeans
1 tsp salt
sprinkling black pepper
½ tsp mild chilli powder
200g (7oz) canned chopped tomatoes
4 garlic cloves, crushed
juice of ½ a lemon
handful of parsley, roughly chopped

Sauté the onion and cinnamon in the oil, then add the beans, salt, pepper, chilli powder and 400ml (14fl oz/1¾ cups) water. Bring to the boil, then simmer for 15 minutes. Add the tomatoes, garlic and lemon juice and simmer for 5 minutes. Serve garnished with parsley.

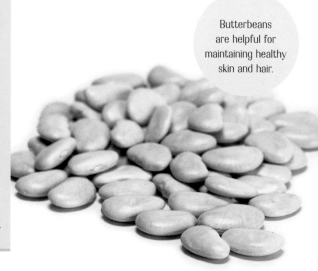

Chickpea

Chickpeas are grown from the equatorial tropics to the temperate northern latitudes of Russia, and are among the most nutritious of pulses.

Chickpeas are a good source of isoflavones, which mimic oestrogen in the body. They can therefore help to prevent hormone-related conditions, including PMS and breast cancer. Chickpeas have antiseptic properties and are a diuretic, making them useful for cystitis and oedema.

They also aid the absorption of nutrients and are good for general digestive health. In addition, chickpeas support the functions of nerves and muscles in the body.

PROPERTIES/ACTIONS
- Mimics oestrogen
- Antiseptic
- Diuretic

PARTS USED
- Whole pulse

HUMMUS

225g (8oz) canned chickpeas
4 garlic cloves, peeled
4 tbsp tahini
4 tbsp olive oil
2 lemons, cut in half

Drain the chickpeas and place them in a food processor, together with the garlic, tahini and olive oil. Squeeze the juice from the lemons and add to the mixture. Blend until pale and creamy. Top with a little olive oil, and serve as a dip with vegetable crudités.

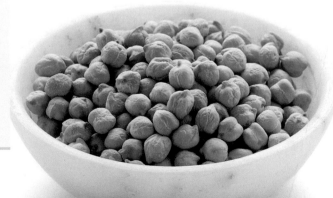

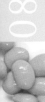

Edamame

NUTRIENTS
Vitamins A, C, folic acid (folate); calcium, iron; omega-3 essential fatty acids

Snacking on edamame, loaded with protein, iron, carbohydrates and fibre, provides a serious stamina boost.

Edamame, which look like a cross between broad beans (fava beans) and peas, are baby soya beans prepared in the pod. Hailed as the latest superfood, the pods are picked while still young and tender. Very popular in Japan, China and Korea, where they have been eaten for hundreds of years, edamame are high in fibre, bone-friendly protein and slow-releasing carbohydrates to help prevent mood fluctuations by keeping blood-sugar levels steady.

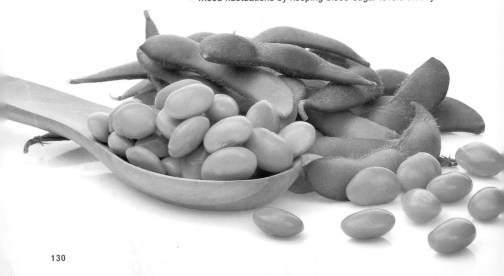

Soya beans have a low glycaemic index (GI) and are great blood sugar and insulin regulators, which makes them useful in maintaining energy levels and for diabetics. They are also a valuable source of B-complex vitamins, which support the nervous system and help to combat stress.

ROASTED EDAMAME BEANS

1 tsp chilli powder
¼ tsp ground cumin
¼ tsp ground coriander
¼ tsp ground ginger
¼ tsp ground turmeric
pinch of paprika
2 tsp sunflower oil
400g (14oz/2 cups) ready-to-eat edamame pods

In a small bowl, mix the spices with the oil. Toss the beans in the mixture and place on a baking tray. Bake in a pre-heated oven at 190ºC/375ºF/Gas 5 for 10–15 minutes. Allow to cool. Serve as a snack.

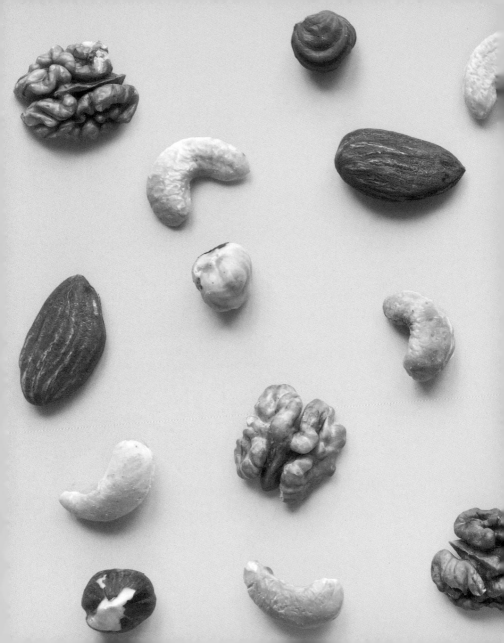

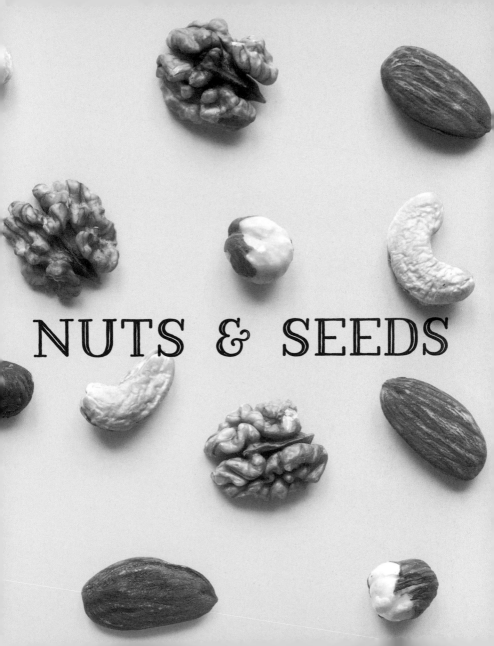

NUTS & SEEDS

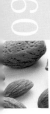

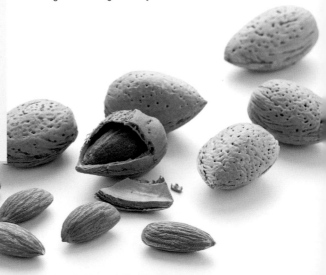

Almond

PROPERTIES/ACTIONS
- Promotes healthy digestion
- Heart protective
- Anti-cancer

PARTS USED
- Whole nut

ALMOND & RAISIN MILK

225g (8oz/2 cups) whole
    almonds (not roasted or
    salted)
handful of dried raisins

Cover the almonds with water
and soak for 24 hours; drain
and rinse. Soak the raisins in
water for 2 hours; drain. Put the
almonds, raisins and 455ml
(16fl oz/2 cups) water in a food
processor. Blend, then strain
through a fine sieve. Keep in the
refrigerator for up to 4 days.

Steeped in history, these sweet, versatile nuts have a higher dietary fibre and calcium content than any other nut and help us to stay healthy.

Due to their relatively high fibre content, almonds help promote healthy digestion, while the calcium in them contributes to strong bones. Almonds also contain the phyto-chemicals quercetin and kaempferol, which may protect against cancer. With over 65 per cent monounsaturated fats that help lower blood fat levels, and a high vitamin E content, almonds can keep LDL cholesterol from oxidizing and sticking to artery walls.

Hazelnut

NUTRIENTS
Vitamins B1, B3, B6, E, folic acid (folate); iron, calcium, magnesium, manganese, potassium; omega-9 fatty acids; protein

Hazelnuts contain an amino acid that can activate cold sores, so avoid them if you are prone to these blisters.

Dense in healthy oils as well as tasty, hazelnuts make a nutritious snack.

Hazelnuts are particularly high in healthy omega-9 fatty acids. They also contain good levels of antioxidant vitamin E, which helps to protect the body from the effects of pollution and other toxins, and vitamin B6, which is needed to make cysteine, a key amino acid for the immune system. Hazelnuts are also rich in important minerals, including iron and calcium, and they are a good source of essential protein.

HAZELNUT BUTTER *makes 1 small bowl*

300g (10½oz/2¼ cups) hazelnuts
2 tbsp sunflower oil
1 tsp raw cane sugar, to taste

Put the shelled nuts on a roasting tray and place in a hot oven to cook for 20 minutes or until the skins crack. Remove from the oven. Rub the skins off with a rough cloth, then place them in a blender with 1 tbsp of the oil. Whizz until a chunky paste forms, then add the remaining oil and the sugar. Blend again until smooth.

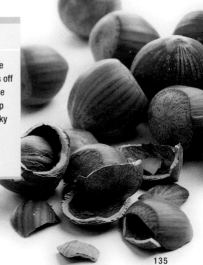

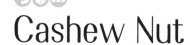

Cashew Nut

NUTRIENTS

Vitamins B2, B3, B5, B6, biotin, folic acid (folate); iodine, iron, magnesium, manganese, potassium, selenium, zinc; protein

These seeds of the Brazilian "cashew apple" are full of healthy fats that can lower cholesterol.

Cashew nuts are a rich source of B-vitamins, which aid the maintenance of the body's nerves and muscle tissue, and boost resistance to stress. They also contain minerals important for immune health, including the antioxidant selenium, which is crucial in the production of antibodies, and virus-fighting zinc, which helps to keep cancer cells at bay. In addition, cashews contain mono-unsaturated fats – these have been shown to help keep cholesterol levels down.

Cashew nuts are a good source of protein, making an ideal snack to stave off hunger pangs.

SUMMER BERRIES WITH CASHEW CREAM *serves 4*

150g (5½oz/1¼ cups) cashew nuts, shelled
1 tsp ground nutmeg
2 tbsp runny honey
200g (7oz/1¾ cups) raspberries
200g (7oz/2 cups) strawberries, hulled and halved

Blend the nuts and 100ml (3½fl oz/7 tbsp) water in a food processor until smooth, then add the nutmeg and honey and whizz again until thoroughly blended. Divide the berries into four bowls, top with the cashew cream and serve.

Walnut

These subtly flavoured nuts are full of nutrients.

Walnuts contain glutathione, an important antioxidant that aids the development of lymphocyte immune cells. They are rich in alpha-linoleic acid (an omega-6 fatty acid) which helps reduce cholesterol levels and boost heart health, and their B-vitamins can provide energy and improve brain function. Their high vitamin E content also makes them a good choice for maintaining healthy skin.

NUTRIENTS
Vitamins B1, B2, B3, B5, B6, E, folic acid (folate); calcium, iron, selenium, zinc; glutathione; omega-6 and -9 fatty acids

Eating just 25g (1oz) of walnuts a day provides half your daily quota of essential alpha-linoleic acid.

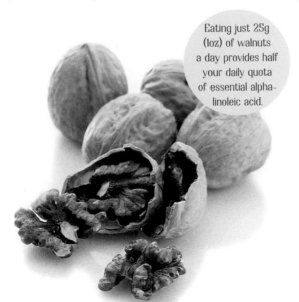

WALNUT PASTA SALAD
serves 4

4 tbsp walnuts, chopped
350g (12oz) wholemeal pasta
  spirals, cooked
3 large tomatoes, cut into
  wedges
handful of rocket (arugula)
2 tbsp chopped basil
1 garlic clove, crushed
4 tbsp walnut oil
2 tbsp balsamic vinegar

In a large bowl, combine all the ingredients except the garlic, oil and vinegar. Whisk these remaining ingredients together, then drizzle over the salad. Serve immediately.

Peanut

Peanuts and peanut butter are packed with protein and heart-healthy fats – a great source of energy for exercise and sports.

In spite of their name, peanuts aren't a nut, but a legume. They're loaded with protein (20–30 per cent) to help muscles stay strong and have a low GI, which means they help to keep blood-sugar levels stable.

LOWER CHOLESTEROL

On the heart-health front, peanuts contain vitamin E, the amino acid arginine and oleic acid (the monounsaturated fat found in olive oil), all of which have been shown to reduce high cholesterol levels in

NUTRIENTS

Vitamins B3, E, folic acid (folate); calcium, copper, magnesium, manganese, phosphorus, potassium

PEANUT FACTS

• Researchers have found that roasting peanuts can increase the level of a compound called p-coumaric acid, increasing their overall antioxidant content by up to 22 per cent.

• The potassium in peanuts helps to regulate the body's water levels and the normal metabolism of food, which prevents cramping, especially during a workout.

• To retain the optimal health benefits, opt for peanut butter made from peanuts only, with no added sodium, sugar or hydrogenated oil.

• Peanuts are one of the foods most commonly associated with allergic reactions.

PEANUT SQUARES

200g (7oz/1¼ cups) roasted
   peanuts
1 tbsp chunky peanut butter
100g (3½oz/½ cup) golden
   granulated sugar
1 tsp bicarbonate of soda
   (baking soda)
1 tsp cornflour (cornstarch)

Finely grind the peanuts in a blender. In a large bowl, mix them with all the remaining ingredients. Press into a small, greased baking tray. Bake at 160°C/315°F/Gas 2–3 for 25 minutes. Cool, cut into squares and serve.

the blood and to protect against the formation of plaque in the arteries, which clogs them up.

FIGHT DISEASE

Peanuts also contain 30 times more resveratrol than grapes – resveratrol is one of a class of compounds called phytoalexins, associated with reduced cardiovascular disease.

Peanuts grow underground, which is why they're often referred to as groundnuts.

INDONESIAN-STYLE PEANUT SAUCE

115g (4oz/⅔ cup) peanuts
juice and zest of 1 lime
250ml (9fl oz/1 cup)
 coconut milk
1 tbsp tamarind paste
1 tbsp curry powder
6 spring onions (scallions),
 finely chopped
chicken, to serve

Blend the peanuts and lime juice and zest in a blender to form a paste. Transfer to a pan and stir in the remaining ingredients and 125ml (4fl oz/ ½ cup) water. Cook over a gentle heat for 7 minutes. Serve over chicken.

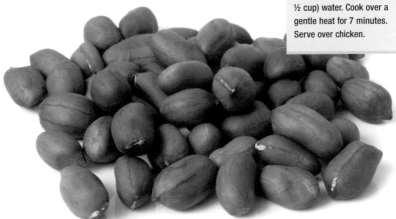

Coconut

NUTRIENTS
Vitamins B1, B2, B3, B5, B6, C, E, folic acid (folate); calcium, copper, iodine, iron, magnesium, manganese, phosphorus, potassium, selenium, zinc

Easily digested and metabolized by the body, coconut is a great pre-exercise energy source.

Although coconut is high in saturated fats known as medium-chain fatty acids (MCFAs), these don't pose the same negative health risk as other saturated fats. This is because the body uses them as instant energy rather than storing them as fat. The coconut water – the liquid inside the coconut – is known to be one of the most balanced natural electrolyte sources, making it a wonderfully rehydrating drink after intensive exercise.

COCONUT RICE

225g (8oz/1 cup) brown rice
1 onion, chopped
1 tbsp ground coriander
1 tbsp ground cumin
2 tbsp coconut oil
2 beef tomatoes, chopped
3 tbsp desiccated (dried shredded) coconut

Place the rice and 500ml (17fl oz/2 cups) water in a pan and bring to the boil. Reduce the heat and simmer for 45 minutes. In another pan, fry the onion and spices in the oil for 3 minutes. Add the tomato and coconut, and simmer for 10 minutes. Mix well with the rice. Serve as a side dish.

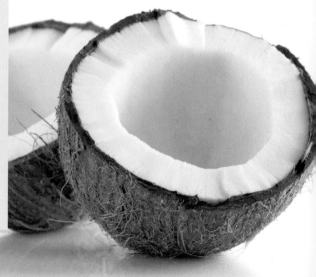

Pine Nut

Full of protein and minerals, these aromatic kernels can aid the prevention of disease.

As well as being rich in the immunity-boosting antioxidant mineral zinc, pine nuts contain high levels of anti-inflammatory polyunsaturated fats, which help to maintain low cholesterol and promote a healthy heart. They are high in vitamin E, which helps protect against the damage that can be caused by pollution and other toxins, and is needed by the immune system's antibodies to fight disease. Pine nuts are also a good source of magnesium, which helps to calm allergic reactions.

Pine nuts can be sprinkled into salads and stir-fries to add a protein kick.

NUTRIENTS
Vitamins B1, B2, B3; E; iron, magnesium, manganese, zinc; protein

RED PEPPER BRUSCHETTA *serves 4*

4 red (bell) peppers, deseeded and sliced
1 garlic clove, crushed
1 tbsp balsamic vinegar
5 tbsp olive oil
1 wholemeal loaf, sliced thickly
200g (7oz) goats' cheese
55g (2oz/½ cup) pine nuts, toasted

Grill (broil) the peppers until soft, then place in a bowl and toss with the garlic, vinegar and 4 tbsp of the oil. Drizzle the remaining oil over the bread, and place in a hot oven to bake until golden on each side, turning once. Top each slice with goats' cheese, peppers and pine nuts.

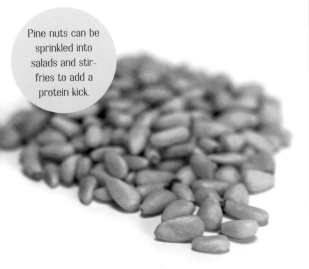

Brazil Nut

NUTRIENTS

Vitamins B1, E, biotin; calcium, iron, magnesium, selenium, zinc; omega-6 fatty acids; glutathione, fibre, protein

High in the antioxidant mineral selenium, the Brazil is one of the most nutritious of all nuts.

The Brazil nut grows wild in the Amazonian rainforest, where it was sacred to ancient tribes. It is the kernel of a fruit that loosely resembles a coconut, and the nuts grow in clusters of up to 24 within this shell. When ripe, the shells fall to the ground. The kernels are then removed, dried in the sun and washed before being exported.

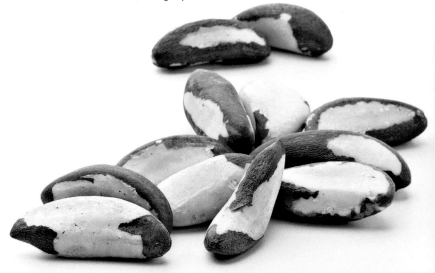

BRAZIL NUT'S IMMUNITY-BOOSTING PROPERTIES

This nut is one of the best sources of selenium, an antioxidant mineral that strengthens the immune system's antibody response and helps to prevent cancer, heart disease and premature ageing. It is a key component in the action of glutathione, an enzyme that suppresses free radicals and helps to halt the development of tumours. Brazil nuts are packed with vitamin E, which works with selenium to provide a super-boost to the immune system. They also contain other important minerals, including magnesium and iron, and are rich in omega-6 fatty acids – essential for easing inflammation in the body, enhancing digestion and improving the skin.

USING BRAZIL NUTS

Rich in protein, a handful of Brazil nuts eaten raw makes a satisfying snack. They can be processed into nut milk or butter, and can be used in stir-fries and salads to add a crunchy protein kick.

BRAZIL NUT FACTS

• Brazil nuts are a vital source of income to the population of the Amazonian rainforest, from where they are most commonly exported to Europe and North America.

• The Brazil nut is also known as the para nut, cream nut (because of its rich flavour) and castanaea.

• After Brazil nuts have been collected, the fibrous, woody capsules that contain the kernels are used as animal traps.

• Brazil nuts have a high fat content, so will turn rancid very quickly and should not be stored for long periods. As with all nuts and seeds, they are best stored in the fridge.

GREEN BEAN AND BRAZIL NUT STIR-FRY *serves 4*

2 tbsp sesame oil
1 onion, chopped
1 tbsp grated fresh ginger
2 garlic cloves, crushed
200g (7oz) asparagus spears
200g (7oz) green beans
100g (3½oz/¾ cup) Brazil nuts, sliced

2 tbsp soy sauce

Heat the sesame oil in a wok over a high heat until it is sizzling hot, then add the onion, ginger and garlic. Stir-fry for 2 minutes, then add the asparagus spears, green beans and Brazil nuts. Continue to stir-fry for a further 5 minutes, then add the soy sauce. Reduce the heat and cook slowly until the asparagus and beans are tender – this should take 8–10 minutes. Serve immediately on a bed of brown rice.

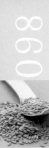

⬡ ♥ 💧 ♨

Sesame Seed & Oil

NUTRIENTS
Vitamins B1, B2, B3, E; calcium, iron, zinc; omega-6 and -9 fatty acids

These tiny seeds can add both taste and essential nutrients to a variety of sweet and savoury dishes.

Sesame seeds have a nutty flavour and are slightly crunchy in texture to eat. Valuable health-boosters, they are made into a number of products such as sesame oil, which is highly resistant to rancidity, and tahini, a sesame-seed paste. Rich in immunity-fortifying zinc and antioxidant vitamin E, they also contain B-vitamins to support the nervous system and to help the body cope with stress. A good source of vegetarian protein, sesame seeds are packed with omega-6 fatty acids for healthy skin and circulation.

> Add sesame seeds to salads and smoothies for a protein boost.

CRUNCHY SESAME STIR-FRY *serves 4*

3 tbsp olive oil
25g (1oz/3 tbsp) sesame seeds
25g (1oz) piece fresh ginger, peeled and grated
2 garlic cloves, crushed
½ a head of broccoli, broken into small florets
3 carrots, cut into long thin slices
½ cabbage, shredded

In a wok, heat the oil and sesame seeds until the seeds start to toast. Then add the ginger and garlic, followed by the other ingredients. Combine well. Turn the heat down to low and fry for a further 5–10 minutes. Serve.

Linseed

Delicate with pretty blue flowers, soothing linseed is wonderful for rehydrating dry skin.

Make a poultice of linseed by adding boiling water to the crushed seeds and stirring the mixture into a paste. Apply the poultice to shingles, psoriasis or burns to soothe away the pain. Or, add a few drops of linseed oil to your bathwater simply to soften your skin. In a tea linseed will soothe a dry, hacking cough. It is a gentle laxative so excellent for overcoming constipation – add a few seeds to a bowl of porridge. The oil is a good source of essential fatty acids, which help support the nervous, immune and hormonal systems.

PROPERTIES/ACTIONS
- Demulcent
- Antitussive
- Laxative
- Emollient
- Expectorant
- Detoxifying
- Anti-inflammatory

PARTS USED
- Ripe seeds (immature seeds can cause poisoning as they contain traces of prussic acid)

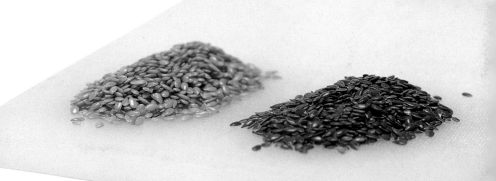

Pumpkin Seed

PROPERTIES/ACTIONS
- Promotes prostate health
- Fights fatigue
- Aids memory

PARTS USED
- Whole seed

Pumpkin seeds are nature's nutritious snack food, supplying plenty of zinc, iron, protein, essential fatty acids and B-complex vitamins.

Due to their high zinc content, pumpkin seeds have a reputation as a male sexual tonic and can reduce an enlarged prostate gland. They also provide a valuable source of energy through the presence of digestible iron.

Containing omega-3 fatty acids, pumpkin seeds are good for the skin and help boost memory-retentive cells. They may help to fight cardiovascular and immuno-deficiency disorders, and are useful in the treatment of intestinal parasites.

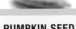

PUMPKIN SEED PORRIDGE

300g (10½oz/1½ cups) pumpkin seeds, unpeeled
500–750ml (16–24fl oz/2–3 cups) milk
honey, to taste

Grind the pumpkin seeds in a food processor or mill. Add 2 cups of milk and blend to form a porridge consistency. Add additional milk, as desired. Transfer to a saucepan and bring to the boil. Add honey to taste, and serve.

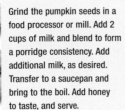

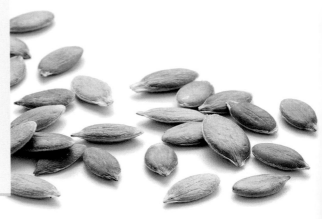

Sunflower Seed

Power-packed with a whole host of nutrients, sunflower seeds are one of the finest energy "pick-me-ups" that nature provides.

Sunflower seeds are a valuable source of B vitamins, which means they are nourishing to the adrenal glands and thus may help to combat energy slumps and many symptoms associated with stress.

The seeds' essential fatty acid content may be beneficial in treating eczema, as well as depression and irritability. Sunflower seeds are a diuretic and expectorant, and have been used in the treatment of bronchial, throat and lung infections.

Native Americans ground sunflower seeds to a meal for thickening soups and drinks.

PROPERTIES/ACTIONS
- Energizing
- Anti-stress
- Diuretic
- Expectorant

PARTS USED
- Whole seed

SEED TRAIL MIX

80g (2¾oz/½ cup) sunflower seeds
40g (1½oz/¼ cup) pumpkin seeds
30g (1oz/¼ cup) blanched almonds, finely chopped
90g (3¼oz/1 cup) flaked and toasted coconut
160g (5¼oz/½ cup) chopped dried apricots

Bake the seeds and nuts on a baking tray at 180°C/350°F/Gas 4 for 4–5 minutes, until golden. Mix with the coconut and apricots.

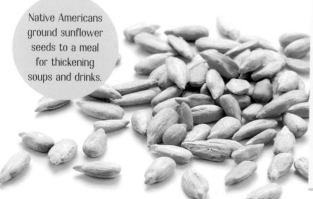

Flaxseed

With abundant and balanced levels of essential fatty acids, flaxseed is acclaimed in history for its ability to prevent and combat many conditions.

Today, the amazing health-giving virtues of flaxseed are recognized throughout the world.

High in both omega-3 and omega-6 essential fatty acids (EFAs), flaxseeds are involved in systematic energy production, oxygen transfer and transportation of fats, and may therefore help to maintain the body's tissue cells, reproductive organs, glands,

PROPERTIES/ACTIONS
- Rich source of EFAs
- Involved in energy production
- Good for reproductive health
- Expectorant

PARTS USED
- Whole seed

FLAXSEED POULTICE

for inflammation, congestion & pain

**2 tbsp ground flaxseed
linen cloth**

Bring the flaxseed and 455ml (16fl oz/2 cups) water to the boil in a pan, then reduce the heat and stir until a thick paste forms. Spread onto the linen cloth and fold this over the paste. Apply the poultice to the affected area. Fix by wrapping another piece of cloth around it. To retain the heat for longer, wrap with a blanket.

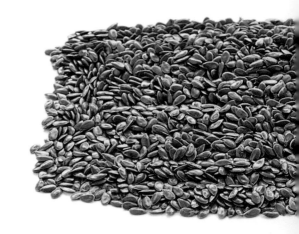

muscles and eyes. Flaxseed is thus traditionally used to treat everything from malnutrition and skin diseases, to arthritis, PMS and fertility problems. Essential fatty acids are also needed to make prostaglandins, hormone-like substances responsible for stamina, circulation and metabolism. Flaxseed can therefore help to maintain healthy blood fat levels and prevent cardiovascular disease.

The ancient Abyssinians were probably the first humans to use flaxseeds for food.

Flaxseed is expectorant and dissolving by nature and may help to treat conditions such as coughs and bronchitis, as well as other inflammatory ailments. The seeds also have a mild purgative action and can be capable of tonifying the bowel, easing constipation.

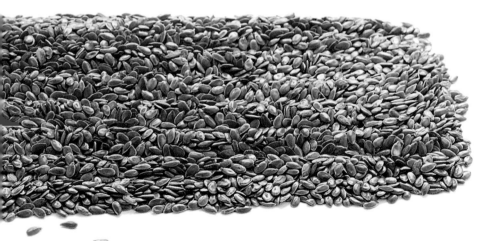

Pistachio

These easy-to-open, pale green nuts are heart-smart and help to maintain good eyesight.

NUTRIENTS

Vitamins B1, B3, E; calcium, copper, magnesium, manganese, potassium, zinc; omega-6 essential fatty acids

Pistachio nuts are known as the "smiling nut" in Iran and the "happy nut" in China.

PISTACHIO FACTS

• The pistachio nut is a member of the cashew family.

• Pistachio trees are planted in orchards, and take up to ten years to produce a significant amount of nuts.

• One serving of pistachio nuts (about 45 kernels) provides as much potassium as half a banana.

• Pistachio nuts contain seven amino acids.

Cardiovascular health and fitness is important, and studies show that eating 25g/1oz of monounsaturated fat-loaded pistachio nuts a day decreases the incidence of heart disease between 20 and 60 per cent.

STRENGTHENS BONES

Pistachios are a good choice because they're also packed with the minerals essential for optimum fitness. Calcium keeps the bones strong; copper increases energy, protects joints and helps the body to utilize iron; magnesium combats muscle fatigue; and zinc speeds up recovery from muscular injuries.

PISTACHIO AND MANGO LASSI *serves 1*

½ mango, peeled and chopped
3 tbsp plain bio-yogurt
55g (2oz/½ cup) pistachios, shelled
2 tsp caster (granulated) sugar

Blend the mango, yogurt, nuts, sugar and 125ml (4½fl oz/ ½ cup) water in a food processor. Serve over ice.

PROTECTS EYESIGHT

Pistachios are also the only nuts that contain high levels of lutein and zeaxanthin, antioxidants needed to maintain eye health.

PISTACHIO COUSCOUS

250g (9oz/1½ cups) couscous
4 cardamom pods, crushed
1 tsp salt
handful of mint
115g (4oz/heaped 1 cup)
   pistachios, shelled
½ tsp grated nutmeg

Bring 500ml (17fl oz/2 cups)
water to the boil in a pan.
Reduce the heat, add the
couscous, cardamom, salt
and mint, and simmer for
10 minutes. Remove from the
heat, fork through the nuts,
add the nutmeg and serve.

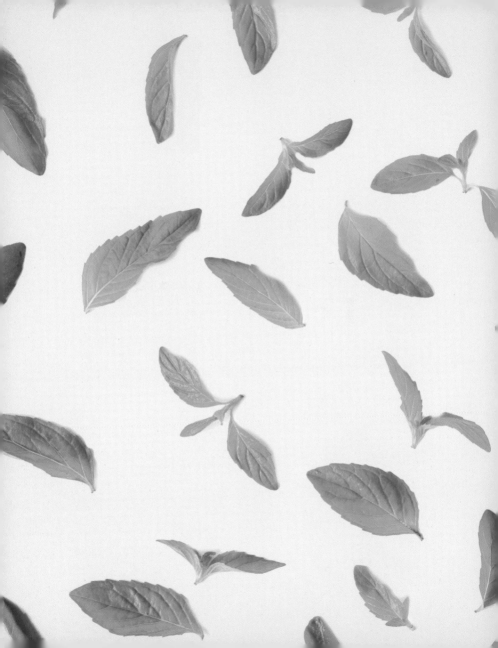

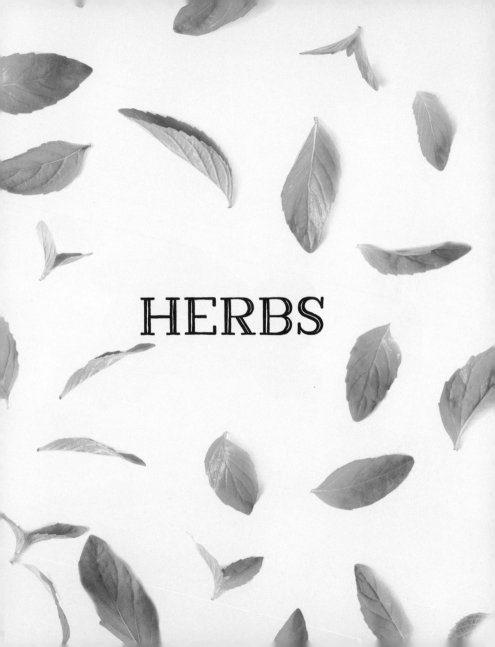

HERBS

Liquorice

Liquorice has a wealth of healing properties, and the Chinese have been using this herb in traditional medicine for thousands of years.

PROPERTIES/ACTIONS
- Lowers stomach acid
- Expectorant
- Anti-arthritic
- Aspirin-like effect

PARTS USED
- Root

Liquorice is a good remedy for lowering stomach-acid levels, so it may help to relieve over-acidity in the digestive tract and stomach ulcers. With its expectorant properties, it is useful for coughs, asthma and chest infections. The root contains glycyrrhizic acid, which gives the herb its anti-inflammatory, anti-allergenic and anti-arthritic actions. With an aspirin-like effect, it is helpful in relieving fevers and headaches. It also acts on the liver, increasing bile flow and lowering cholesterol.

Alexander the Great, Caesar and Brahma endorsed the properties of liquorice.

LIQUORICE INFUSION
for coughs & chest complaints

**25g (1oz) liquorice root
1 heaped tsp flaxseeds
110g (4oz/⅔ cup) raisins
110g (4oz/⅔ cup) brown sugar
1 tbsp white wine vinegar**

Place the liquorice, flaxseed, raisins in a saucepan with 2 litres (70fl oz/8¾ cups) water, and bring to the boil. Leave to simmer until the water has reduced by about half. Add the sugar and white wine vinegar, then stir well. Drink 240ml (8fl oz/1 cup) before going to bed.

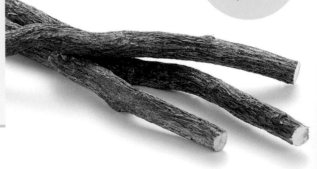

Hops

**Hops – a much-loved flavouring in beer –
will ease away tension, anxiety and pain.**

Hops can calm the nervous system and are wonderful for reducing problems related to stress. A nervous system that is out of kilter can affect the healthy functioning of the digestive system. Hops will help to impede this link, while stimulating digestion and liver function. The stress-busting effects reach our muscles, too: the plant's antispasmodic properties relieve muscle tension. Regular cups of hop tea are both diuretic and detoxifying; while the estrogenic effects of hops make them great for relieving symptoms of the menopause.

PROPERTIES/ACTIONS
- Sedative
- Relaxant
- Antispasmodic
- Bitter tonic
- Digestive
- Astringent
- Diuretic
- Estrogenic
- Painkilling
- Antiseptic

PARTS USED
- Dried strobiles of the female plant

Hops can act as a mild depressant. Avoid them if you suffer from depression.

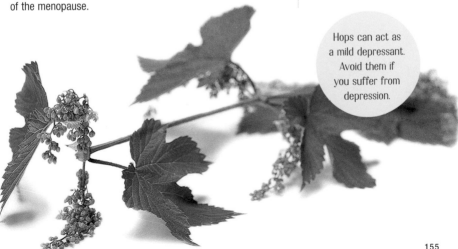

Elecampane

PROPERTIES/ACTIONS
- Expectorant
- Antitussive
- Diaphoretic
- Antimicrobial
- Antiseptic
- Bitter tonic
- Cholagogue
- Anthelmintic
- Digestive

PARTS USED
- Rhizomes

A stately plant with bright yellow flowers, bitter elecampane will hasten away chest infections.

Before the advent of antibiotics, doctors often treated pneumonia and tuberculosis with elecampane. Antifungal, antibacterial and expectorant, this wonderful herb will see off catarrh, colds, asthma, bronchitis, whooping cough, and other chest infections. The herb also stimulates digestion, regulates the bowels, and helps expel toxins from the body. Hot elecampane tea will bring down a fever; cooled, the tea makes a great antiseptic wash for wounds and cuts, and for skin infections such as scabies and herpes.

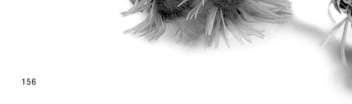

Fennel

PROPERTIES/ACTIONS
- Anti-spasmodic
- Diuretic
- Combats fluid retention
- Aids digestion

PARTS USED
- Seed

FENNEL & CLOVE MOUTHWASH

½ tsp fennel seeds
½ tsp ground cloves
2 tbsp pure grain alcohol or good-quality vodka
250ml (9fl oz/1 cup) distilled water
paper coffee filter

In a bowl, mix the spices into the alcohol. Cover and leave for 3 days, then pour through the coffee filter placed in a strainer. Add the water. Store in a sealed bottle for 6 weeks. Gargle with 1 tbsp at a time, as a mouthwash.

Part of the parsley family, the fennel plant and seeds have ancient medicinal properties and are also popular culinary ingredients.

Fennel is well known for its anti-spasmodic, analgesic and diuretic properties. It can be used to ease digestive problems, combat fluid retention and reduce intestinal spasms. Because it aids elimination of toxins through the urine, it is also a useful remedy for arthritis and gout. Its volatile oils have antiseptic effects, particularly useful for urinary infections.

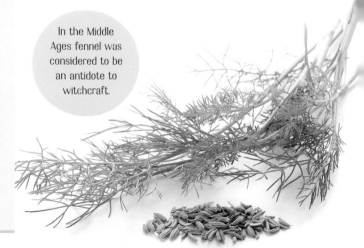

In the Middle Ages fennel was considered to be an antidote to witchcraft.

Cleavers

PROPERTIES/ACTIONS
- Diuretic
- Alterative
- Anti-inflammatory
- Astringent
- Antitumour
- General tonic
- Refrigerant
- Mild laxative

PARTS USED
- Aerial parts

A common hedgerow weed, cleavers is a wonderful cleanser and detoxifier.

Our ancestors ate cleavers' soup to lose weight, but today cleavers is used mainly as a cleansing remedy to clear toxins and reduce heat and inflammation. Soothing and diuretic, cleavers is also good for cystitis, fluid retention, arthritis and gout, and taken regularly as tea can help to clear myriad skin conditions. If you have swollen lymph nodes (glands), cooling cleavers can help to reduce congestion and inflammation; it will also reduce fevers. Apply an infusion of cleavers to burns and abrasions, and as a hair rinse against dandruff.

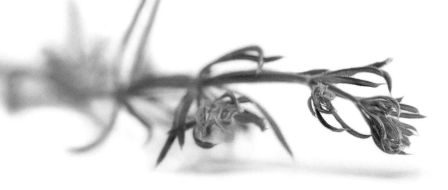

Echinacea

Also known as purple coneflower, there are various species of echinacea, all of which have been therapeutically effective throughout history.

Known as a non-specific immuno-stimulant, this herb has been shown to increase white blood cell count and promote respiratory cellular activity. It is used for colds, influenza, ear infections, chronic fatigue and allergies. Its anti-viral properties appear to be due to the stimulation of interferon-like effects. Traditionally, echinacea has also been used to promote healing and reduce inflammation, both internally for conditions such as colitis, and externally for ailments such as acne.

PROPERTIES/ACTIONS
- Immuno-stimulant
- Helps colds & influenza
- Promotes healing

PARTS USED
- Root

ECHINACEA THROAT DECOCTION

20g (¾oz) dried or 40g (1½oz) fresh echinacea root

Place the echinacea root in a saucepan, cover with 750ml (24fl oz/3 cups) water and bring to the boil. Simmer for about 20–30 minutes, until the liquid has reduced by about one-third. Strain through a sieve into a jug. Discard the echinacea. Gargle about 50ml (1¾fl oz) of liquid, either hot or cold, 3 times a day. Store in a cool place for up to 3 days.

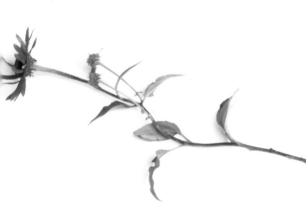

Boneset

PROPERTIES/ACTIONS
- Diaphoretic
- Febrifuge
- Aperient
- General tonic
- Antispasmodic
- Peripheral vasodilator
- Alterative
- Cholagogue
- Mild laxative
- Expectorant
- Decongestant

PARTS USED
- Aerial parts of the flowering plant

A member of the hemp family, boneset is the perfect antidote to the first signs of flu.

Boneset encourages circulation to your muscles to relieve the aches and pains that herald the onset of flu, helps throw off fevers, and clears congestion. Rheumatism and similar muscular pains also respond well to boneset. Its laxative effects can help to ease constipation. Boneset can also treat skin conditions linked with poor liver function. Recent research indicates that the herb may help fight cancer as it contains lactones that may prevent secondary tumours, and flavones, which encourage the healthy functioning of cells.

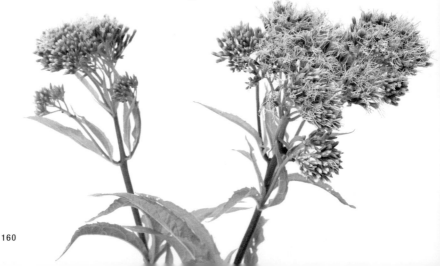

Limeflower

PROPERTIES/ACTIONS

- Nervine
- Antispasmodic
- Diaphoretic
- Diuretic
- Mild astringent
- Hypotensive
- Peripheral vasodilator

PARTS USED

- Flowers

Also known as the linden flower, honey-scented limeflower comes from a tree loved by bees.

Symbolizing female beauty and grace, the linden tree gives us the perfect antidote to stress and stress-related illness, including headaches, tension and irritability. Taken as a tea, sweet-tasting limeflower helps to calm restlessness and induce sleep. If you suffer from coronary problems, limeflower can relax the arteries, ease palpitations and reduce high blood pressure. The cooling properties of limeflower tea will help to chase away a fever. Apply the tea externally to ease the pain of burns and scalds.

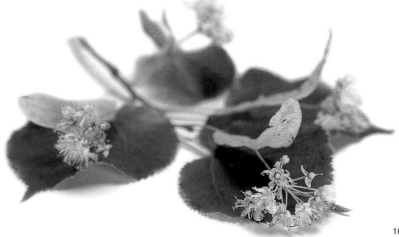

112

Rosehip

NUTRIENTS
Vitamin C, carotenoids; fibre

Packed with vitamin C, this little seed pod can be highly effective in staving off colds and 'flu.

Rosehips are actually the seed pods of roses and appear on rose bushes after they have flowered. They contain twenty times more vitamin C than oranges by weight and therefore help to improve resistance to infections, such as the common cold, by enhancing the cleaning action of phagocytes (white blood cells) and detoxifying bacteria. Rosehips are also a good source of pectin, a type of fibre that binds to cholesterol and toxins to carry them out of the body.

ROSEHIP SYRUP

125g (4½oz) rosehips
125g (4½oz/heaped ½ cup) raw
cane sugar

Place the rosehips and 500ml (17fl oz/2 cups) water in a saucepan, bring to the boil, then leave to cool. Strain through a muslin (cheesecloth) several times to remove seeds, sharp fibres and pulp. Bring the strained liquid back to the boil, add the sugar and simmer until the volume is reduced by about a third. Cool and pour into a small sterile bottle.

During World War II, children in Britain were given rosehip syrup to prevent vitamin C deficiency.

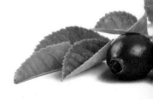

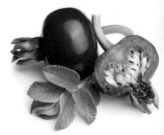

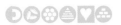

Red Clover

Give yourself a spring clean with this deeply cleansing, wild herb with its cheerful red flower.

Red clover is diuretic and mildly laxative, helping to clear wastes through both the urinary and digestive systems. It also stimulates the liver, the body's built-in detoxifier. The flower is completely safe to give to both adults and children to help to ease conditions such as eczema and asthma. Red clover may be able to inhibit the growth of tumours, especially in female cancers, such as ovarian or breast cancer. It is also good for menopausal women: it helps to balance hormones and reduce symptoms such as hot flushes.

PROPERTIES/ACTIONS
- Alterative
- Expectorant
- Antispasmodic
- Relaxant
- Diuretic
- Anti-inflammatory
- Hormone-regulating
- Antitumour
- Antiviral
- Antifungal
- Cholesterol-lowering
- Detoxifying
- Immune-boosting

PARTS USED
- Flowers

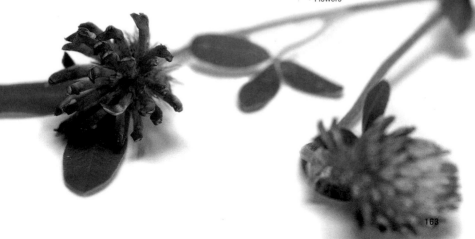

163

Eyebright

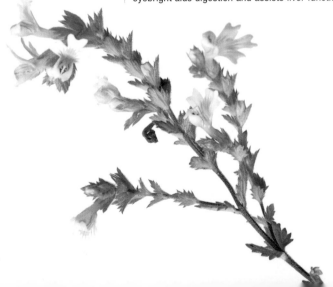

PROPERTIES/ACTIONS

- Astringent
- Anti-inflammatory
- General tonic
- Decongestant
- Digestive
- Cholagogue
- Alterative

PARTS USED

- Leaves
- Flowers

With its pretty white flowers that look like eyes, eyebright is the best remedy for eye problems.

An eyebright decoction is wonderful as a tea, but also makes an eyewash or a soak for a compress to treat myriad eye irritations. Whether you suffer from light-sensitivity, a stye, conjunctivitis, or blepharitis, eyebright will help to reduce inflammation and soothe sore eyes. Its anti-inflammatory and decongestant properties make it great for treating upper respiratory tract conditions, for relieving nasal congestion, sinusitis, hay fever, and colds. As a bitter tonic, eyebright aids digestion and assists liver function.

Meadowsweet

PROPERTIES/ACTIONS
- Astringent
- Antacid
- Stomachic
- Anti-emetic
- Antirheumatic
- Anti-inflammatory
- Antiseptic
- Diuretic
- Diaphoretic
- Painkilling

PARTS USED
- Aerial parts of the flowering plant

Queen of the meadow, this herb is the natural equivalent of aspirin – without the side-effects.

Meadowsweet will protect and soothe the lining of the digestive tract, making it the perfect remedy for all digestive conditions, from heartburn to ulcers. Meadowsweet contains salicylates, crystals of salicylic acid, that help to reduce inflammation in arthritis, rheumatism and gout, and soften deposits, such as kidney stones and any build-up in the arteries. Take it as a hot tea to reduce fevers and the aches and pains of flu; and to relieve headaches. Externally, apply a soothing cooled meadowsweet tea to inflamed skin or eyes.

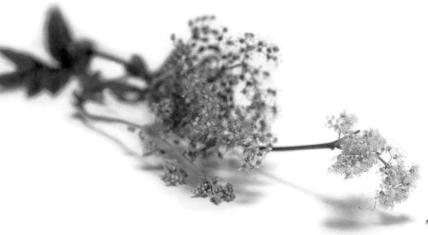

Peppermint

A well-known digestive aid, peppermint has many other benefits and is one of the most popular traditional remedies used today.

PROPERTIES/ACTIONS

- Soothes digestive tract
- Protects gut lining
- Improves circulation
- Decongestant
- Analgesic
- Antiseptic

PARTS USED

- Leaves

Peppermint soothes the digestive tract, and is used for heartburn, indigestion and nausea. It improves the circulation, and can help chills, fevers, colds, influenza, stuffiness and congestion. The herb also has analgesic properties, which are useful for headaches, inflamed joints, neuralgia and sciatica. The volatile oils have antiseptic properties, and are antibacterial, anti-parasitic, anti-fungal and anti-viral.

PEPPERMINT FOOT BATH
for tired feet

**50g (2oz/2½ cups) peppermint leaves, roughly chopped
1 litre (35fl oz/4 cups) boiling water
1.75 litres (60fl oz/7½ cups) hot water
1 tsp borax
1 tbsp Epsom salts**

Combine the herbs with the boiling water in a large bowl. Leave for 1 hour, then strain. Add to a bowl or footbath filled with the hot water. Stir in the borax and Epsom salts. Soak the feet for 15–20 minutes.

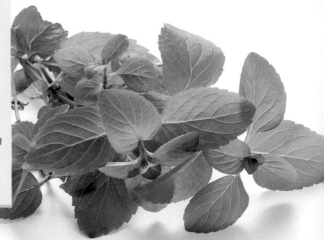

Basil

Sweet basil can refresh you when you feel tired, and calm you when you feel tense or anxious.

If you are feeling stressed and exhausted, and suffering any of the related symptoms (headaches, indigestion, muscle tension, nerve pain, and so on), or you feel that your concentration or memory need a boost, basil will provide the tonic. The herb is both antiseptic and cleansing, helping the body to overcome all manner of infections. Hot basil tea reduces fevers and clears phlegm from the chest and nose, and so eases the symptoms of colds, flu, catarrh, coughs and sore throats. Its relaxant properties extend to both the digestive and respiratory tracts, and can relieve colic, constipation and nausea, and ease conditions such as asthma and tight coughs.

PROPERTIES/ACTIONS
- Carminative
- Sedative
- Stomachic
- Antibacterial
- Anthelmintic
- Anti-depressant
- Antispasmodic
- Adrenal stimulant
- Febrifuge
- Diaphoretic
- Decongestant
- Peripheral vasodilator

PARTS USED
- Leaves

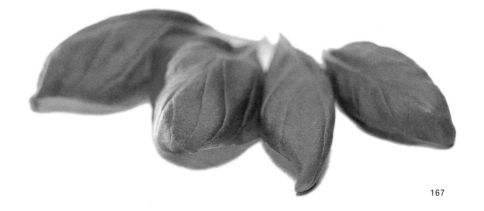

★⊕♥⊛

Rosemary

PROPERTIES/ACTIONS

- Astringent
- Anti-spasmodic
- Invigorating
- Nervine

PARTS USED

- Leaves

TONIC WINE & LINIMENT
for stiff muscles, headaches, etc

handful of rosemary leaves
2 small cinnamon sticks
5 cloves
1 tsp ground ginger
a bottle of good-quality red
wine

Lightly crush the rosemary, cinnamon and cloves in a tall jar, using a pestle. Add the ginger, then the wine, seal the jar and leave in a cool place for 7–10 days. Strain and store in a sealed bottle. Drink a glass daily, or dip a cotton-wool pad and apply to the affected area.

A potent, stimulating herb, rosemary is an old-fashioned remedy for everything from colds and colic, to nervousness and eczema.

Rosemary has antiseptic, antioxidant, anti-spasmodic and astringent qualities, proving useful for circulatory conditions, stiff muscles, coughs and colds, mouth and gum infections, and irritable bowel syndrome.

An invigorating herb, rosemary fights fatigue. It is also a nervine and is excellent for female complaints and headaches. The essential oil can be used as an insect repellent.

Used in shampoos, rosemary is also reputed to prevent premature baldness.

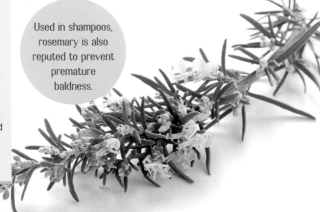

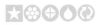

Sage

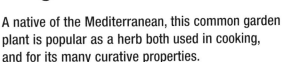

PROPERTIES/ACTIONS
- Treats respiratory conditions
- Decongestant
- Digestive aid
- Calming & soothing

PARTS USED
- Leaves

A native of the Mediterranean, this common garden plant is popular as a herb both used in cooking, and for its many curative properties.

With its fragrant aroma, sage has antiseptic, antibacterial and anti-viral properties, and is a traditional ingredient of cough, cold and respiratory remedies. With decongestant and astringent effects and an ability to reduce mucus, it is particularly successful in the treatment of bronchitis.

Sage stimulates the intestines and is a tonic for the digestive system. It also clears sluggish skin and firms tissues, is calming and soothing, and fights emotional distress.

SAGE & THYME GARGLE

for respiratory ailments

large handful of sage leaves
small handful of thyme leaves
450ml (16fl oz/2 cups) boiling water
2 tbsp cider vinegar
2 tsp honey
1 tsp cayenne pepper

Roughly chop the leaves and place in a jug. Add the water, cover and leave for 30 minutes. Strain off the leaves and stir in the vinegar, honey and cayenne. Gargle with the mixture at the first sign of symptoms, or drink 2 tsp 2 or 3 times a day. Use within a week.

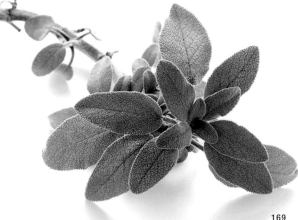

Elder & Elderflower

The elder tree is truly a pharmacy in itself, providing medicines for all manner of illness. Traditionally known as "nature's medicine chest", the elder tree provides both flowers and berries with medicinal properties.

PROPERTIES/ACTIONS
- Expectorant
- Circulatory stimulant
- Depurative
- Diuretic
- Anti-inflammatory
- Diaphoretic
- Laxative
- Decongestant
- Antioxidant
- Immuno-stimulant
- Induces sweating
- Diuretic
- Treats respiratory conditions

PARTS USED
- Flowers
- Berries

Both the flowers and berries induce sweating and dispel toxins, clearing heat and inflammation from the body. The flowers alone are decongestant, anti-inflammatory and relaxant, and excellent for colds, flu and catarrh. The leaves, flowers, berries and bark are all diuretic. Elderflower has a well-established reputation as an

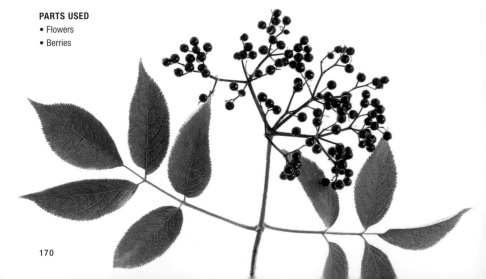

ELDERFLOWER SALVE

for dry, chapped skin

150g (5½oz) emulsifying wax
70g (2½oz) glycerine
30g (1oz) dried or 75g (2½oz)
  fresh elderflower tops

Melt the wax in a glass bowl set
in a pan of boiling water. Stir in
the glycerine, herbs and 80ml
(2½fl oz/⅓ cup) water. Simmer
for 3 hours, then pass through
a strainer lined with muslin
(cheesecloth). Stir until cool and
set. Transfer to dark glass jars
with lids. Rub into the affected
area 3 times a day. Store in the
refrigerator for up to 3 months.

immune stimulant and for fighting coughs and colds. It can induce
perspiration, and is useful in the treatment of fevers. By acting as
a diuretic, elder flowering tops aid the removal of waste products
and are valuable in arthritic conditions. They also tone the mucous
linings of the nose and throat, increasing resistance to conditions
such as asthma, bronchitis, sinusitis and hayfever. Elderflowers
contain ursolic acid, which has an anti-inflammatory action and
can soothe chapped skin. Elderberries are rich in immune-boosting
vitamin C, and have a laxative effect.

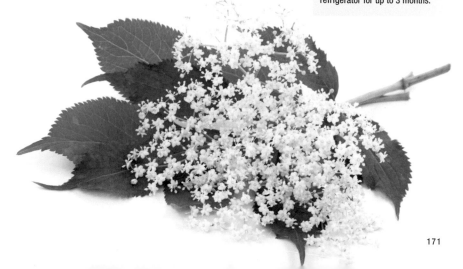

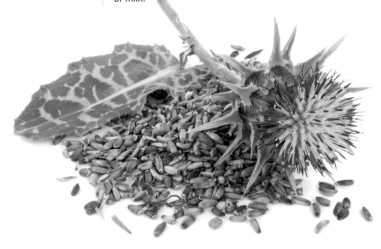

Milk Thistle

PROPERTIES/ACTIONS
- Cholagogue
- Galactagogue
- Demulcent
- Immune-boosting
- Detoxifying

PARTS USED
- Seeds

If you live your life in the fast lane, protect your body with some nurturing milk thistle.

Headaches, early-morning lethargy, poor digestion of fatty foods, and dark, thick menstrual blood may all be signs that your liver is under pressure. Milk thistle is able to enhance the function of the liver and even regenerate liver-tissue, making it essential for anyone who has sustained liver damage, whether through disease (such as hepatitis), alcohol abuse, pollution or stress. The gall bladder is known to benefit, too. The plant is perfectly safe for breast-feeding mothers, who can use it to increase their flow of milk.

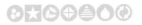

Yarrow

A summer herb, found wild in the countryside, yarrow is renowned as a remedy for bleeding.

PROPERTIES/ACTIONS
- Diaphoretic
- Febrifuge
- Peripheral vasodilator
- Hypotensive
- Anti-allergenic
- Vulnerary
- Emmenagogue
- Styptic
- Anti-inflammatory
- Astringent
- Diuretic
- Digestive
- Urinary antiseptic
- Decongestant
- Hormone-regulating
- Detoxifying

PARTS USED
- Aerial parts of the flowering plant

Yarrow's astringent properties have a drying effect on body fluids and help to stem blood-flow, curb diarrhea and clear catarrh. The herb is also great to stimulate the appetite, enhance digestion and absorption, and relax tension in the gut. Antiseptic and anti-inflammatory, yarrow speeds healing in gastritis and enteritis. A hot tea can overcome fevers, colds and flu, and a lukewarm or cold tea relieve cystitis. Use yarrow tea externally to bathe wounds, varicose ulcers and burns, as well as hemorrhoids, and skin conditions such as eczema.

Avoid taking yarrow during pregnancy.

Dandelion

PROPERTIES/ACTIONS

- Diuretic
- Blood purifier
- Treats liver
- Increases bile production
- Rich in iron

PARTS USED

- Whole herb

With healing properties in the roots, leaves and flowers, dandelion is a faithful folk remedy and one of the most frequently prescribed herbs.

Dandelion leaves are a powerful diuretic and are useful for bladder infections and oedema. The roots are a blood purifier, helping to remove toxins from the liver and kidneys. The leaves and roots produce mannitol, which is used for hypertension and a weak heart. An appetite stimulant, dandelion increases production of bile to help relieve digestive ailments. Rich in vitamins and iron, it is also useful for treating anaemia.

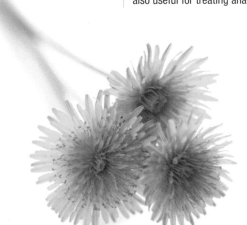

DANDELION TONIC WINE

60g (2¼oz/1 cup) dandelion
   flowers
1 litre (35fl oz/4 cups)
   white wine
honey, to taste

Crush the flowers using a pestle and mortar, then place them in an airtight container. Pour in the white wine, seal the container and steep for 1 month, then strain out the flowers. Sweeten with honey, if desired. Drink 1 cup.

Eucalyptus

PROPERTIES/ACTIONS
- Expectorant
- Soothing
- Antiseptic
- Anaesthetic effect

Warning: eucalyptus should not be used by people with liver disorders or digestive problems.

PARTS USED
- Leaves

Best known for its expectorant properties, the Australian plant eucalyptus is nature's own remedy for respiratory conditions.

Eucalyptus can soothe the mucous membranes, making it a suitable herb for chest infections. It also clears the nasal passages, and has antiseptic properties that are helpful for colds, influenza and sore throats. The essential oil protects from insect bites, and when used as a chest or sinus rub, it has a warming and slightly anaesthetic effect. It may relieve stiffness in rheumatic joints, and help bacterial skin infections.

EUCALYPTUS DECONGESTANT RUB *for colds, blocked noses, etc*

50g (2oz) petroleum jelly
1 tbsp dried lavender
6 drops eucalyptus
    essential oil
4 drops camphor essential oil

Melt the petroleum jelly in a bowl over a pan of simmering water. Stir in the lavender and heat for 30 minutes. Strain the jelly through a piece of muslin (cheesecloth) and leave to cool slightly. Add the oils. Pour into a jar and leave to set. Rub into the chest, throat or back, depending on symptoms.

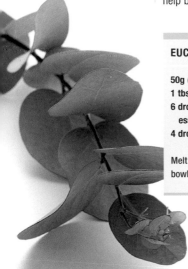

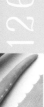

Aloe Vera

PROPERTIES/ACTIONS
- Soothes skin conditions
- Treats digestive problems
- Anti-cancer

PARTS USED
- Sap & leaves

This herb belongs to the lily family, and its leaves provide a sap that has unique anti-inflammatory and healing properties.

Aloe vera is used most commonly for helping the healing of burns, wounds and skin irritations. When prepared as a juice, it may aid conditions such as colitis, stomach ulcers, kidney stones and constipation. It is rich in nutrients and has been used traditionally for treating everything from fluctuating blood-sugar levels to hangovers. More recently, it has been recognized for its cancer-fighting potential.

Aloe vera was first valued by the ancient Egyptians as a medicinal plant.

ALOE VERA JUICE
for stomach disorders

5 large aloe vera leaves

Pulp the leaves, preferably using a mechanical juicer. Squeeze the pulp through a strainer lined with a muslin (cheesecloth) to collect the juice. Drink during symptoms.

Marsh Mallow

Soothing marsh mallow is wonderful for all kinds of irritation and inflammation.

Marsh mallow contains an abundance of mucilage, which coats and protects the lining of the respiratory, digestive and urinary tracts. Its expectorant properties mean that marsh mallow can soothe dry coughs, sore throats, and bronchitis. The plant will also relieve inflammatory digestive problems, such as heartburn and gastritis, and urinary problems, such as cystitis. Rub the leaves on the affected area to soothe insect bites, scalds, sunburn and rashes. A warm poultice will draw out splinters; a mouthwash will soothe sore gums.

PROPERTIES/ACTIONS
- Emollient
- Demulcent
- Vulnerary
- Anti-inflammatory
- Mild expectorant
- Diuretic
- Immune-boosting
- Painkilling

PARTS USED
- Roots
- Leaves
- Flowers

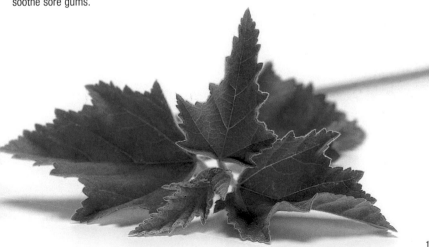

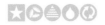

Burdock

This handsome plant draws toxins out of the body, making it a wonderful cleanser.

PROPERTIES/ACTIONS

- Bitter tonic
- Digestive
- Diuretic
- Diaphoretic
- Laxative
- Antimicrobial
- Alterative
- Hypoglycemic
- Anti-inflammatory
- Detoxifying

PARTS USED

- Roots
- Leaves
- Seeds

Burdock has the ability to absorb toxins from the gut and carry them through to the bowel for elimination; its diuretic properties clear toxins via the kidneys. A great liver remedy, the plant can relieve inflammatory conditions such as arthritis and gout, and inflammatory skin problems such as eczema and psoriasis. As an effective antibacterial and antifungal herb, burdock will fight all manner of infection. Apply the poultice externally to ulcers, bruises, sores and boils; and the decoction to impetigo, cold sores and ringworm.

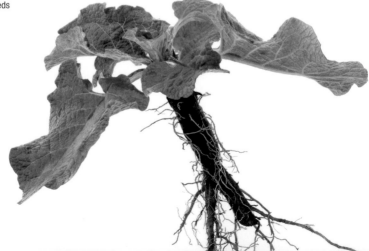

Calendula/Marigold

PROPERTIES/ACTIONS
- Relaxant
- Alterative
- Astringent
- Antiseptic
- Antimicrobial
- Antispasmodic
- Anti-ulcer
- Anti-inflammatory
- Antitumour
- Antioxidant
- Antihistamine
- Diaphoretic
- Diuretic
- Bitter tonic
- Digestive
- Cholagogue
- Detoxifying
- Estrogenic
- Vulnerary

PARTS USED
- Flowers

Avoid taking marigold in any form during pregnancy.

This cheerful, golden flower takes pride of place as an antiseptic, first-aid remedy.

Marigold enhances immunity and helps the body fight bacterial, fungal and viral infections. In the digestive tract it relieves irritation and inflammation and aids digestion and nutrient-absorption. Taken as a hot tea, marigold brings down fevers, improves blood and lymphatic circulation, and regulates menstruation. In the uterus it clears the congestion that contributes to period pain, excessive bleeding, fibroids and cysts. Apply marigold externally to soothe cuts, sores, skin problems, varicose veins, warts, burns, and cold sores.

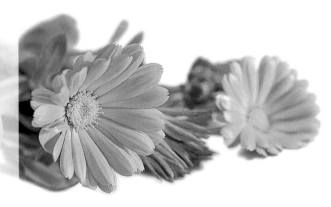

Gotu Cola

PROPERTIES/ACTIONS

- Nervine
- Cardiac tonic
- Immune-boosting
- Febrifuge
- Alterative
- Diuretic
- Antiseptic
- Anthelmintic
- Vulnerary
- Rejuvenative
- Hair tonic
- Anticonvulsant
- Anxiolytic
- Analgesic
- Anti-inflammatory
- Painkilling
- Circulatory stimulant

PARTS USED

- Leaves

A wonderful brain tonic, gotu cola boosts our brain power and keeps us young.

Gotu cola aids memory and concentration and has proved excellent in helping children with autism and learning difficulties, including ADHD (attention deficit hyperactivity disorder). It relieves stress, anxiety, insomnia and depression, and soothes indigestion, acidity and diarrhea, and helps to clear skin problems. By stimulating healing in the connective tissue, gotu cola helps wounds knit together and reduces scarring. Apply the oil to your head and feet at night to prevent insomnia, or rub it into your scalp to prevent early balding and greying in your hair.

Gota cola is known as the "herb of longevity".

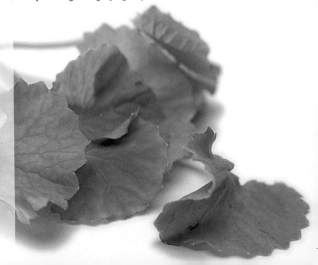

Ginseng

PROPERTIES/ACTIONS
- Increases vitality
- Prevents nervous disorders
- Treats digestive troubles
- Aphrodisiac

PARTS USED
- Root

GINSENG SOUP

2 carrots, sliced
2 celery sticks, chopped
2 medium potatoes, peeled and
   chopped
1 onion, chopped
1 tbsp olive oil
4g (⅙oz) dried ginseng root
½ tsp salt
½ tsp black peppercorns

Sweat the vegetables in oil in
a large pan for 5–6 minutes.
Add the other ingredients along
with 2 litres (70fl oz/8¾ cups)
water. Bring to the boil, then
simmer for 2 hours, skimming
occasionally. Whizz in a blender.
Check the seasoning and serve.

Discovered some 5,000 years ago in the mountain provinces of China, *panax ginseng* is a useful nutritive tonic and general stimulant.

Ginseng is well known for its ability to increase energy and vitality. It raises body metabolism and is believed to increase the utilization of nutrients and oxygen in the cells. It also slows the heart rate and decreases the heart's demand for oxygen, and prevents nervous disorders such as anxiety and stress.

Studies show an improvement in cognitive ability with daily usage. Ginseng also treats stomach and digestive troubles, lowers blood-sugar levels and is said to prolong longevity.

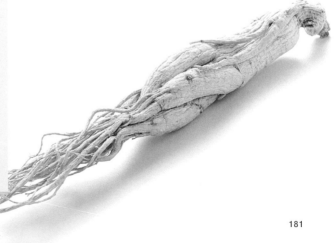

Garlic

NUTRIENTS

Vitamin B6; iron, magnesium, phosphorous, selenium, zinc; amino acids, volatile oils

An ingredient few cooks would be without, this pungent bulb has many therapeutic properties.

Widely used in cooking throughout the world, garlic is thought to have originated in central Asia. It was used in ancient Egypt and Greece, where it played a role in rituals as well as being an important medicinal food. Traditionally garlic was used to fight a range of diseases, from gastro-intestinal conditions to respiratory infections.

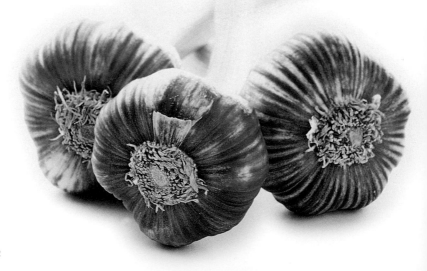

GARLIC'S IMMUNITY-BOOSTING PROPERTIES

Garlic is a potent anti-microbial, boosting the production of white blood cells and fighting off bacteria, parasites, fungi and viruses. These properties make it a useful weapon against conditions from yeast infections to food poisoning and the common cold. Garlic helps boost heart health by actively lowering cholesterol levels, and allicin, a volatile oil found in the bulb, may help suppress the formation of tumours. It is also a powerful antioxidant, thanks to its amino acids, helping it to enhance overall immune function.

USING GARLIC

Versatile and tasty, garlic can be added to virtually any savoury dish to boost its flavour – add one clove per person for its full health-boosting effects. It gives a kick to stir-fries, casseroles and sauces, and can be chopped and added raw to salads and dressings. Garlic can also be taken in supplement form.

GARLIC FACTS

• Be careful not to eat an excess of garlic if you are taking medication to combat high blood pressure, as garlic can exaggerate the effects of the drugs.

• Fresh parsley can help to eradicate the strong smell of garlic on the breath.

• Garlic's sulphur compounds can irritate gastric ulcers.

• Garlic bulbs keep best stored in a cool, dry place. If the air is too damp they tend to sprout, and if it is too warm the cloves eventually turn to grey powder.

TOMATO, BASIL AND GARLIC SALAD *serves 4*

800g (1lb 12oz) large ripe
  tomatoes, sliced
4 tbsp roughly chopped basil
2 garlic cloves, finely chopped
6 tbsp olive oil
2 tbsp balsamic vinegar
sea salt and black pepper

Arrange the tomatoes flat on a large plate, and sprinkle over the remaining ingredients. Serve immediately.

Comfrey

PROPERTIES/ACTIONS
- Heals tissue, bone & cartilage
- Treats skin complaints

Warning: comfrey should not be used internally, or on open wounds.

PARTS USED
- Leaves & root

An ancient wayside plant of the borage family, comfrey is native to Britain and Russia, and is a useful first-aid remedy.

Cultivated since 400BCE, comfrey is one of the most famed healing plants. With the traditional name of "knitbone", it has remarkable powers to heal tissue, bone and cartilage, and was used for these purposes by the Greeks and Romans.

Comfrey's renowned healing ability is due to the presence of a compound called allantoin, which promotes cell proliferation and encourages ligaments and bones to knit together firmly. Allantoin is easily absorbed through the skin, making comfrey a very effective herb for topical use. Comfrey has the ability to reduce swellings and can help to heal injuries including fractures. This herb also

---

COMFREY BRUISE OINTMENT

200g (7oz) petroleum jelly or paraffin wax
30g (1oz/½ cup) roughly chopped comfrey leaves

Bring a saucepan of water to the boil. Put the jelly or wax into a glass, heat-proof bowl, and place the bowl over the pan of water. Reduce the heat so that the water is simmering, then add the chopped leaves to the jelly or wax and continue to simmer for about an hour. Remove the bowl from the heat and strain the mixture through a muslin (cheesecloth). Pour immediately into a glass jar and allow to set. Use the ointment as needed.

treats many other skin conditions including psoriasis, eczema and varicose veins, as well as sprains and bruises. Traditionally known as "bruisewort", recent American research has also shown that comfrey breaks down red blood cells, a finding that supports its use for bruises. Comfrey is also valuable in the treatment of scars.

There is some debate on the safety of internal consumption of this herb due to the fact that it contains pyrrolizidine alkaloids which are believed to be toxic to the liver.

Comfrey was known to the ancient Greeks for its amazing ability to make new tissue.

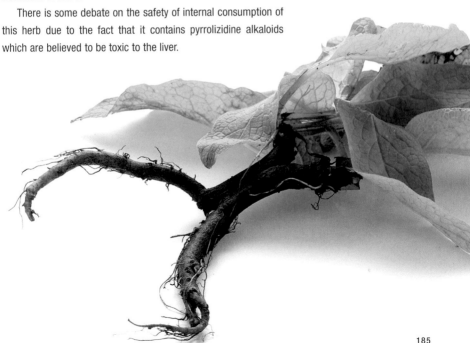

Black Cohosh

PROPERTIES/ACTIONS
- Oestrogenic action
- Alleviates menstrual problems
- Benefits rheumatic & arthritic conditions
- Nervine

PARTS USED
- Root

Black cohosh is a Native American remedy long used for women's ailments, especially those associated with menopause.

Black cohosh has an oestrogenic action, and is thought to reduce levels of pituitary luteinizing hormone. This makes it useful for alleviating menstrual problems and reducing menopausal hot flushes. Black cohosh also has anti-inflammatory properties, which benefit rheumatic and arthritic conditions. Its expectorant qualities make it useful for asthma and bronchial symptoms. Due to its sedative effect, it can also treat nerve conditions.

BLACK COHOSH DECOCTION

20g (¾oz/⅛ cup) dried or 40g (1½oz/¼ cup) chopped fresh black cohosh root

Place the herb in a saucepan, cover with 750ml (26fl oz/ 3 cups) water and bring to the boil. Simmer for 20–30 minutes, until the liquid is reduced to about 500ml (17fl oz/2 cups). Using a sieve, strain the liquid into a jug. Allow to cool or drink hot, taking 50ml (1¾fl oz/3½ tbsp) 3–4 times a day. Cover the jug and store in the refrigerator for up to 48 hours.

Slippery Elm

The powdered bark of the elm tree, slippery elm has a long history of use among the Native Americans, who first discovered its distinct strengthening and healing properties.

The mucilage in this herb makes it a soothing remedy for the lining of the stomach, which may help digestive problems such as irritable bowel syndrome, Crohn's disease and colitis. When made into a gruel, it is especially effective for colicky babies. It also soothes sore throats. When used topically, slippery elm disperses inflammation and imparts an emollient effect, thus soothing wounds, burns and itchy, irritated skin.

PROPERTIES/ACTIONS
- Mucilaginous
- Soothes digestive tract
- Eases colic
- Emollient

PARTS USED
- Bark

SLIPPERY ELM SOUP
for the throat & stomach

1 tsp slippery elm powder
1 tsp sugar
455ml (16fl oz/2 cups) boiling water
ground cinnamon, ginger or nutmeg, to taste

Combine the slippery elm, sugar and water, then mix well. Flavour with the cinnamon, ginger or nutmeg, to taste. Drink as symptoms arise. For a creamier texture, you can use milk instead of water.

136

Feverfew

PROPERTIES/ACTIONS
- Treats migraine
- Women's herb
- Lowers temperature

PARTS USED
- Leaves

Feverfew is now used principally as a treatment for migraine, but has long been thought of as a herb for a variety of other ailments.

Although the exact nature of its actions is not yet fully understood, the constituent parthenolide found in feverfew appears to inhibit the release of the hormone serotonin, which is thought to trigger migraine.

Feverfew also has many gynaecological uses for women. With a stimulant effect on the uterus, it can induce menstruation, and with relaxant and analgesic properties it eases period pains. Feverfew can lower temperature and has traditionally been used for hot flushes during menopause.

FEVERFEW TINCTURE

200g (7oz/13 cups) dried or 300g (10½oz/19½ cups) chopped fresh feverfew
1 litre (35fl oz/4 cups) alcohol

Place the herbs and alcohol in a large glass jar. Put the lid on the jar and shake well. Store in a cool, dry place for 10–14 days, shaking the jar every 1–2 days. Strain the herbs from the liquid by pouring it through a piece of muslin (cheesecloth). Discard the herbs. Pour the tincture into a dark glass bottle with a lid. Take 5 drops with water up to 3 times a day.

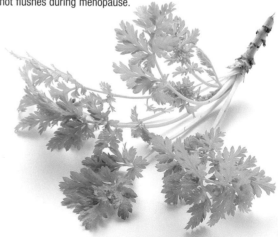

Horseradish

This close relative of mustard can help to fight infection and boost circulation.

NUTRIENTS
Vitamin C; calcium, magnesium, phosphorus; volatile oils

Horseradish has antispasmodic properties, promotes the flow of bile and is particularly good for sinus problems. It is a powerful circulatory stimulant, and also boosts digestion. Its anti-bacterial properties make it a useful cold remedy, while the volatile mustard oil it contains gives it expectorant capabilities, beneficial for loosening catarrh. Its vitamin C content is useful for generally bolstering the immune response.

Avoid horseradish if you have an underactive thyroid.

APPLE AND HORSERADISH SAUCE *makes 1 small bowl*

2 cooking apples, peeled, cored and grated
2 tbsp freshly grated horseradish
juice of 1 lemon
1 tsp salt
2 tsp finely chopped mint

200ml (7fl oz/¾ cup) sour cream or fromage frais

Combine all the ingredients together in a bowl and mix thoroughly. Chill for 1 hour, then serve as an accompaniment to a meat or vegetable dish.

Skullcap

PROPERTIES/ACTIONS
- Nervine
- Sedative
- Antispasmodic
- Mild astringent
- Duretic
- Thymoleptic
- Anti-inflammatory
- Painkilling

PARTS USED
- Leaves
- Flowers

A member of the mint family, pretty skullcap makes an excellent tonic for the nerves.

Skullcap offers support for a busy, stressful life. Soothing and calming, skullcap can ease away anxiety, lift your mood and even relieve depression. If you feel tired or exhausted, skullcap will help to promote restful sleep. Combine skullcap with hormone-balancers, such as vitex, to reduce the symptoms of PMS or the menopause, and to help steady mood swings. The herb is also anti-inflammatory and painkilling. A hot cup of skullcap tea will reduce a fever.

✿★✛○

Thyme

With its pungent scent, thyme has been used by healers for centuries, and today is among the most common and useful of herbs in the garden.

A stimulating herb, thyme works well as a tonic for the nerves, helping to combat mental stress and enhance mood. It has powerful antiseptic, antibacterial and anti-viral actions, and is used for treating respiratory troubles such as asthma, coughs and colds, and allergic reactions. With a local anaesthetic-like effect, thyme has proved useful for tonsillitis. Applied topically, thyme can help heal wounds as well as muscular pain. Thyme also contains strong anti-fungal properties for treating nail fungus, athlete's foot and yeast infections.

PROPERTIES/ACTIONS
- Nervine tonic
- Treats respiratory conditions
- Anaesthetic-like action
- Anti-fungal

PARTS USED
- Leaves

THYME LINCTUS
for disorders of the respiratory tract

25g (1oz) thyme leaves
25g (1oz) borage flowers and leaves
2 small cinnamon sticks
juice of 1 small lemon
100g (3½oz/6 tbsp) honey

Simmer the herbs and cinnamon sticks in 455ml (16fl oz/2 cups) water for 20 minutes. Strain, and return the liquid to the pan. Simmer until reduced by half. Add the lemon juice and honey; simmer for 5 minutes. Take 1 tsp as required.

Nettle

PROPERTIES/ACTIONS
- Nourishing
- Rich in iron
- Dense in chlorophyll

PARTS USED
- Leaves

NETTLE TONIC TEA

40–50g (1½–2oz/½–1 cup) chopped nettle leaves

Put 1 litre (35fl oz/4 cups) water in a saucepan and bring to the boil. Add the nettle leaves to the water, then reduce the heat and simmer for 5–10 minutes. Strain and discard the herbs. Drink 1 cup 3 times a day before meals.

Stinging nettle nourishes the whole system, specifically the adrenals and kidneys, and has long been used as a remedy for rheumatism.

Very high in iron, nettle is a good tonic for blood disorders such as anaemia. The leaves are high in chlorophyll, which acts on the hormonal system, and the root is rich in vitamin C, which boosts immunity and treats conditions such as hayfever.

Nettle is often used to reduce inflammation in allergic responses and rheumatism. It is also a nourishing tonic for pregnant and lactating women.

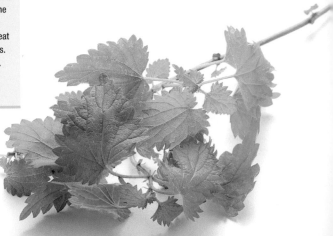

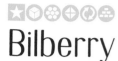

Bilberry

Delicious, blue fruits, bilberries burst with nutrients to keep us young and healthy.

Bilberries contain antioxidants that help to repair environmental damage to our skin, and help to prevent the degenerative symptoms of the ageing process; tannins that help to protect the digestive, urinary and respiratory systems from infection; and vitamins A and C, bioflavonoids, and iron. The fruits are also antiviral and antifungal, and have an antibiotic effect in the urinary tract. Try bilberry juice for a fever or for inflammation; or a bilberry mouthwash for mouth ulcers or a sore throat.

PROPERTIES/ACTIONS
- Antibacterial
- Antiviral
- Diuretic
- Diaphoretic
- Antioxidant
- Astringent

PARTS USED
- Berries
- Leaves

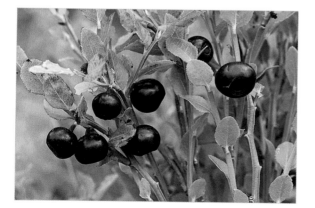

Bilberries can cause allergic reactions in some people.

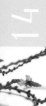

Vervain

PROPERTIES/ACTIONS
- Nervine
- Antidepressant
- Relaxant
- Cholagogue
- Febrifuge
- Galactagogue
- Emmenagogue
- Diuretic
- Antispasmodic
- Anti-inflammatory
- Digestive

PARTS USED
- Leaves
- Flowers

A delicate plant, with pretty mauve flowers, vervain is a great friend in times of stress.

Almost all forms of stress and stress-related symptoms can benefit from vervain's relaxing and mood-lifting properties. If you suffer from PMS, try vervain to lift your spirits and reduce period pain. Vervain is quite a bitter herb and so is good for the digestive system, stimulating the flow of gastric juices and enhancing the absorption of nutrients. It also enhances liver and gall-bladder function. Hot vervain tea can reduce a fever. Taken cool the tea can clear bacteria from the urinary tract, making it a good remedy for cystitis.

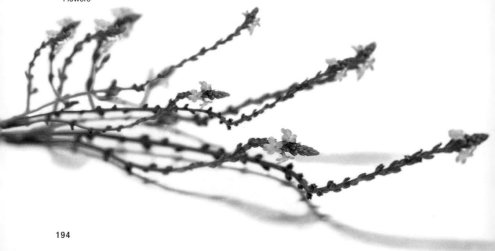

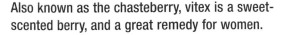

Vitex

Also known as the chasteberry, vitex is a sweet-scented berry, and a great remedy for women.

Vitex has a simply amazing ability to regulate the hormones, making it the best remedy for period pain, PMS, and a range of gynecological complaints, including fibroids, endometriosis, and ovarian cysts. It is also excellent for fertility problems, painful or swollen breasts, and the symptoms of the menopause. In women who are breast-feeding, vitex can help to promote a good supply of milk. In men vitex is often able to cool sexual passion, a property that has given rise to its nickname, "monk's pepper".

PROPERTIES/ACTIONS
- Uterine tonic
- Galactagogue
- Hormone-regulating
- Antispasmodic
- Relaxant

PARTS USED
- Berries

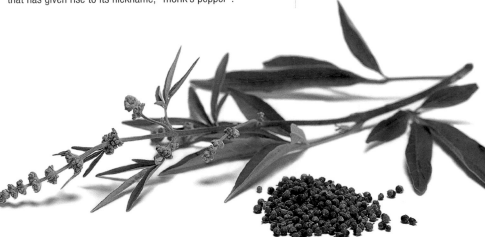

Ashwagandha

PROPERTIES/ACTIONS
- Sedative
- Nervine
- Rejuvenative
- Anti-inflammatory
- Antitumour
- Adaptogen
- Antioxidant
- Immune-boosting
- Painkilling
- Antimicrobial
- Antispasmodic
- Reproductive stimulant

PARTS USED:
- Roots

Known as "Indian Ginseng", Ashwagandha increases energy and induces calm.

Ashwagandha is a must for anyone with a busy, stressful life. Use it to strengthen your reserves and reduce all the telltale signs of stress, such as insomnia and exhaustion. The herb is both rejuvenative and antioxidant, helping to speed recovery from illness. Its sedative properties can help to calm children with behavioural problems. As an immune-booster, ashwagandha can be given in auto-immune diseases such as multiple sclerosis and rheumatoid arthritis.

Both women and men can use ashwagandha to boost fertility and libido.

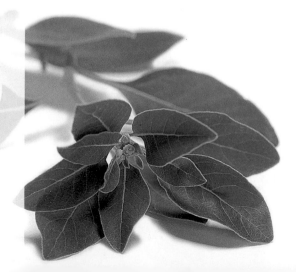

Hawthorn

Part of the rose family, hawthorn came to the attention of the medical profession in the 1890s and became known as the herb for "hearts".

The hawthorn plant has a vasodilatory effect, proving an excellent remedy for high blood pressure and angina. Hawthorn also acts on the vagus nerve, treating mild arrthymia. By increasing circulation to the brain, hawthorn improves memory. It also decreases inflammation caused by allergies, and has a relaxant effect in the digestive tract, relieving intestinal discomfort.

PROPERTIES/ACTIONS
- Vasodilator
- Improves memory
- Relaxes digestive tract
- Treats nervous conditions

PARTS USED
- Flowers & berries

HAWTHORN "HEART" TINCTURE

200g (7oz/1 cup) dried or 300g (10½oz/1½ cups) chopped fresh hawthorn flowers or berries
1 litre (35fl oz/4 cups) alcohol

Place the hawthorn in a large glass jar and cover with the alcohol. Secure the lid and shake. Store in a cool, dark place for 10–14 days, shaking every 1 or 2 days. Strain through a muslin (cheesecloth) into a dark glass bottle. Take 1 tsp 3 times a day in 25ml (1fl oz) water or juice. Store for up to 2 years.

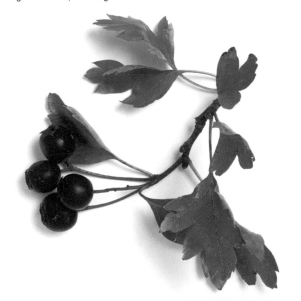

Wild Yam

PROPERTIES/ACTIONS

- Antispasmodic
- Antirheumatic
- Diuretic
- Anti-inflammatory
- Cholagogue
- Relaxant
- Peripheral vasodilator
- Expectorant
- Estrogenic
- Emmenagogue
- Hormone-regulating

PARTS USED

- Roots
- Rhizomes

Wild yam's roots contain substances similar to progesterone, making this the "woman's herb".

Whether you suffer from PMS or menstrual problems, or are going through the menopause, wild yam is one of the best herbs to correct hormonal imbalances. The plant provides a substance called diosgenin, which pharmacists once used in the manufacture of the contraceptive pill to mimic the hormone progesterone and prevent ovulation. Wild yam's antispasmodic properties ease menstrual cramping, muscular spasm, colic, and flatulence. Its anti-inflammatory properties make wild yam a good remedy for arthritis and gout.

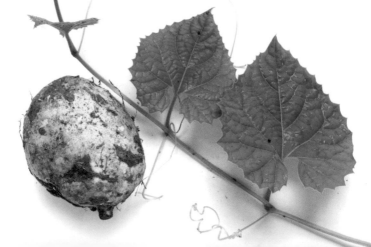

St John's Wort

PROPERTIES/ACTIONS
- Anti-depressant
- Fights colds
- Treats nervous system
- Astringent

PARTS USED
- Flowers

Historically, St John's wort has been used for a number of disorders, but it is best known for its treatment of mild depression.

This herb is said to lend a sunny disposition and is used for depression, anxiety and fatigue, as well as loss of appetite. It is a powerful anti-viral and fights colds, herpes simplex and hepatitis. It is also traditionally used for affections of the nervous system, namely neuralgia and sciatica. As an astringent and diuretic it is useful for inflammatory conditions, particularly those of the urinary tract.

OIL INFUSION
for inflammatory skin conditions

handful of fresh or dried St John's wort flowers
500ml (17fl oz/2 cups) olive oil

Place the herbs in a glass bottle or jar with a stopper, and cover with the olive oil. Drizzle the oil on salads, removing any flowers. Steep until all the oil is used.

199

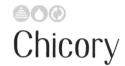

Chicory

Wild chicory enjoys a reputation in traditional medicine as a great spring tonic with powerful cleansing and detoxifying abilities.

Chicory leaves, commonly used in salads, are effective as a liver stimulant. With an amazing ability to promote secretion of bile, chicory treats jaundice and aids the detoxifying process.

Chicory has an equally beneficial effect on the kidneys, and is useful for urinary infections, skin problems, arthritis, rheumatism and gout. It also has anti-inflammatory properties and can settle stomach disorders.

PROPERTIES/ACTIONS
- Liver stimulant
- Good for skin problems
- Helps arthritis
- Settles the stomach

PARTS USED
- Root & leaves

OLD-FASHIONED CHICORY DEPURATIVE SYRUP

1kg (2lb 4oz/6 cups) fresh chicory root
500g (1lb 2oz/2½ cups) granulated sugar

Wash the chicory root thoroughly, then press through a juicer. Place the juice in a saucepan together with the sugar. Bring to the boil, then reduce the heat and simmer for about 20 minutes, until the juice acquires a syrupy consistency. Store in a tightly sealed bottle. Take 1 tsp 1–3 times a day.

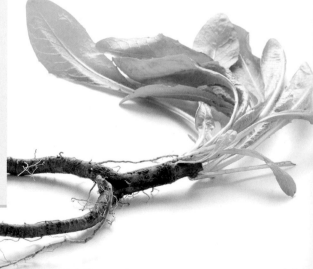

Lavender

This fragrant herb, which adorns our gardens in the spring and has been popular since the Middle Ages, is a unique tonic for the nervous system.

PROPERTIES/ACTIONS
- Soothing
- Treats anxiety & insomnia
- Antihistamine effect

PARTS USED
- Whole herb

LAVENDER COMPRESS
for headaches, burns, bites, etc

15g (½oz/¼ cup) dried or 30g (1oz/½ cup) fresh lavender
250ml (9fl oz/1 cup) vodka
square of cotton cloth

Put the herb in a glass jar with the vodka and 50ml (1¾fl oz/ 3½ tbsp) water. Cover and leave in a cool, dark place for 7–10 days. Strain off the lavender with a sieve lined with a paper towel, and wrap it in the cloth. Apply directly to the affected area. Alternatively, make a liniment by soaking a cotton-wool pad in the tincture and dabbing it onto the skin.

Lavender is a tonic and sedative, and may therefore help anxiety, headaches, insomnia and general stress. It also has antibacterial and antiseptic properties, useful for conditions such as acne, eczema and yeast infections.

Due to its antihistamine properties, inhaling the vapours of lavender essential oil is useful in treating bronchitis, and lavender's prostaglandin-inhibiting effects can help to reduce the pain and swelling of burns and bites. Lavender is also anti-spasmodic and a diuretic.

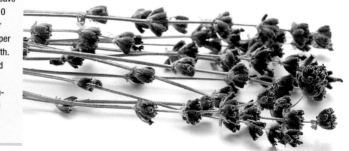

Chamomile

PROPERTIES/ACTIONS

- Carminative
- Sedative
- Antihistamine
- Anti-spasmodic
- Children's remedy

PARTS USED

- Whole herb

STEAM INHALATION

for problematic skin

½ tsp chopped chamomile
  leaves
250ml (9fl oz/1 cup) purified
  water

Simmer the herbs and water
in a saucepan for 30 minutes.
Pour the boiling water and
herbs into a bowl and, keeping
your face within a safe distance
from the water, cover both
your head and the bowl with
a towel and inhale for about
30 seconds. Repeat 2 or 3
times a day.

One of the herbs in the Anglo-Saxon "Nine Herbs
Charm", chamomile has an ancient and detailed
medicinal history.

Chamomile is best known for its calming nervine effects and is
often used to treat anxiety and insomnia, as well as attention deficit
hyperactivity disorder (ADHD). It is also an antihistamine, thus
relieving allergic symptoms, and has anti-inflammatory and antispasmodic properties that help it to treat digestive disorders such
as irritable bowel syndrome, as well as PMS and skin conditions
such as eczema.

Chamomile is an excellent remedy for children's ailments,
including colic and teething.

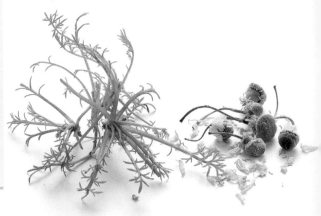

Chickweed

Although the active constituents in chickweed are largely unknown, it is a renowned folk remedy for a number of conditions.

With its demulcent and cooling properties, chickweed is especially useful for the treatment of conditions such as eczema, nappy rash, and even chicken pox. When applied as a compress, it can treat conjunctivitis and ear infections.

Traditional Chinese herbalists use chickweed to treat everything from asthma and indigestion, to nosebleeds and rheumatic conditions.

PROPERTIES/ACTIONS
- Demulcent
- Cooling
- Soothes skin

PARTS USED
- Whole herb

CHICKWEED OIL
for skin & rheumatic conditions

225ml (8fl oz/scant 1 cup) sunflower oil
375g (13oz/6 cups) fresh chickweed (leaves and flowers)

Pour the sunflower oil into a bowl and place it over a large saucepan of boiling water. Add the chickweed. Simmer gently for 2 hours, topping up the water as necessary. Strain the oil into a bottle. Dab the oil directly onto the skin. Alternatively, add 1 tbsp to warm bath water.

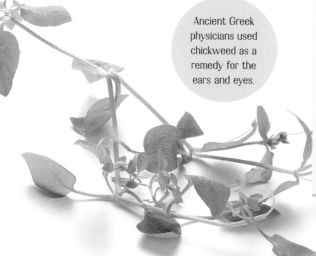

Ancient Greek physicians used chickweed as a remedy for the ears and eyes.

NATURE'S PHARMACY

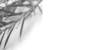

Tea Tree

PROPERTIES/ACTIONS
- Anti-fungal
- Antiseptic
- Treats skin infections
- Useful for oral infections

PARTS USED
- Leaves

Native to Australia, tea tree is part of the clove family and provides one of the most effective natural antiseptics.

With its antibacterial, anti-fungal and renowned antiseptic properties, tea tree is an effective remedy for a broad range of conditions, especially fungal and skin problems like ringworm, insect bites and stings, acne, athlete's foot and yeast infections. Tea tree is effective as a mouthwash, counteracting gum disease, and can also be used as a gargle for sore throats. It is useful as a remedy for coughs and colds.

TEA TREE SKIN WASH

1 tsp dried or 2 tsp fresh tea tree leaves
250ml (9fl oz/1 cup) freshly boiled water

Steep the herbs in the water for 5–10 minutes, then strain. Allow to cool, then bathe the skin or affected area. Repeat when required.

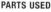

Evening Primrose

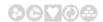

PROPERTIES/ACTIONS
- Astringent
- Anti-inflammatory
- Antispasmodic
- Digestive
- Immune-boosting
- Hormone-regulating
- Expectorant
- Cholesterol-lowering
- Hypotensive
- Anti-allergenic
- Sedative

PARTS USED
- Oil from seeds
- Leaves
- Stems
- Flowers

The elegant evening primrose provides great support for women's hormonal problems.

The oil of the evening-primrose seed contains GLA (gamma linoleic acid), a fatty acid that is vital for healthy functioning of both the immune system and the hormones. Try it if you are menopausal, or suffer from PMS. Evening primrose is also an excellent remedy for arthritis, auto-immune problems, and allergies. This healing herb can help to ease withdrawal symptoms from alcohol dependency and counteract the effects of excess alcohol on the liver. You can take the oil internally for skin problems, such as eczema.

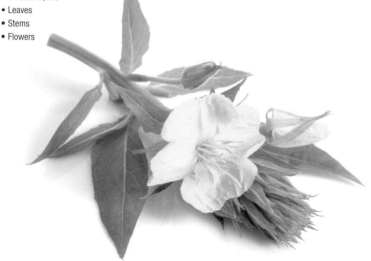

Lemon Balm

PROPERTIES/ACTIONS
- Sedating
- Liver & gallbladder stimulant
- Treats digestive conditions
- Reduces mucus

PARTS USED
- Whole herb

LEMON BALM SALVE

for bruises, bites & cold sores

handful of lemon balm leaves, dried or fresh
250ml (9fl oz/1 cup) almond oil
25g (1oz) beeswax
½ tbsp vitamin E oil

Place the herbs in a glass jar and cover with the almond oil. Leave for 2 weeks, shaking daily, then strain through a piece of muslin (cheesecloth). Melt the beeswax in a pan. Add the oil and mix. Off the heat, add the vitamin E oil. Store in jars in the refrigerator. Apply liberally to the skin.

With a lovely citrus scent, lemon balm has many medicinal, culinary and aromatic uses.

Due to its sedating effects, lemon balm has been used traditionally for treating menstrual cramps and headaches, healing wounds, easing digestion, preventing insomnia and relaxing the nerves. It stimulates the liver and gallbladder, and enhances digestion and absorption. The herb has a particular affinity for easing nausea, colitis, colic and irritable bowel syndrome. It has antibacterial, antiviral and mucus-reducing properties, and is good for children's coughs and colds. Used topically, it can relieve swellings, bruises, bites and cold sores.

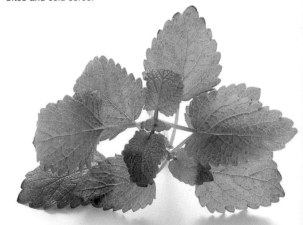

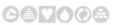

Coriander

PROPERTIES/ACTIONS
- Carminative
- Diuretic
- Decongestant
- Antispasmodic
- Antimicrobial
- Diaphoretic
- Digestive
- Circulatory stimulant
- Refrigerant
- Anti-inflammatory
- Detoxifying

PARTS USED
- Ripe seeds
- Leaves

Once considered an aphrodisiac, coriander is best known as an excellent aid to digestion.

Coriander (cilantro) enhances the appetite and improves the body's absorption of nutrients. The leaves themselves are rich in vitamins A and C, as well as calcium, potassium and iron. The herb has long been known as a tonic for the brain and nerves, and its cooling effects will calm fevers and inflammatory problems, such as cystitis, sore throats, hay fever and arthritis, and reduce hot flushes. Apply the leaves' juice or the tea externally to relieve hot, itchy skin rashes. The tea also makes a great gargle for sore throats and oral thrush.

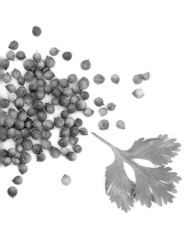

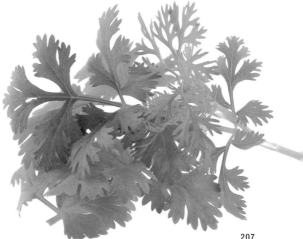

Parsley

PROPERTIES/ACTIONS
- Relaxant
- Antiseptic
- General tonic
- Depurative
- Uterine tonic
- Diuretic
- Digestive
- Nervine
- Antirheumatic
- Antispasmodic

PARTS USED
- Roots
- Leaves
- Seeds

Since ancient times parsley has been used to enhance youth and beauty, and boost libido.

Parsley is packed with nutrients, notably vitamin C, which improves immunity and assists the body's absorption of iron, making this a good herb for anemia sufferers. Parsley stimulates the kidneys, helping to detoxify the body; and soothes the digestive tract, relieving conditions such as colic, indigestion and wind. Use a decoction of the seeds to ease abdominal cramps and headaches. Parsley can stimulate the uterine muscles; avoid it during pregnancy unless you want to use it to enhance contractions during childbirth.

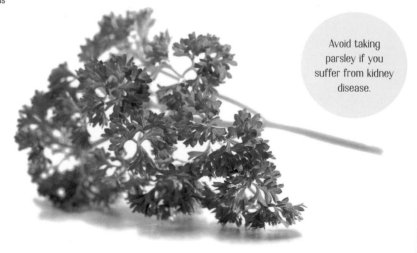

Avoid taking parsley if you suffer from kidney disease.

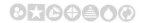

Plantain

This unassuming leaf is great for combating inflammation and allergies.

If you suffer from eczema, acne or boils, plantain leaves will cool inflamed skin and expel toxins. Infections such as colds, sinusitis and earache, and conditions such as hay fever and asthma, respond well to hot plantain tea. The zinc-rich leaves can be helpful for an enlarged prostate, as well as stem bleeding, diarrhea and excessive menstruation. The plant's seeds (psyllium seeds) will bulk out stools, providing an excellent remedy for constipation or irritable bowel syndrome. Crush the fresh leaves as a topical first-aid treatment.

PROPERTIES/ACTIONS
- Anti-inflammatory
- Astringent
- Alterative
- Diuretic
- Vulnerary
- Demulcent
- Refrigerant
- Detoxifying
- Decongestant
- Expectorant
- Antiseptic
- Antispasmodic
- Laxative

PARTS USED
- Leaves
- Seeds

Do not eat the seeds for two hours before and after taking medicine, as they can inhibit absorption.

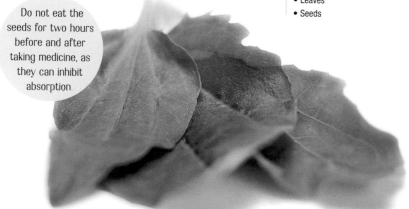

Rose

The beautiful, sweet-smelling rose is the bloom of lovers – and also of well-being and longevity.

Rose leaves and petals can reduce fever, dispel toxins, boost immunity, and rebalance the bacterial population in the gut. If you are anxious, agitated, grieving or suffer from sleep problems, rose hips, petals and oil can all help to calm the mind and body, lift the

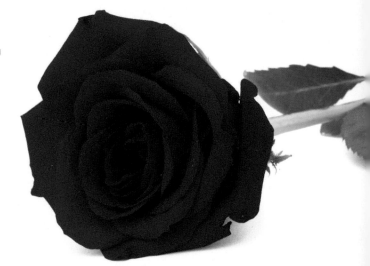

mood, and promote restful sleep. A feminine flower, the rose has a special affinity for women, helping to relieve pelvic congestion and painful or heavy periods, and increase libido. Applied to the skin, rose water is wonderfully toning and cleansing and has powerful antiseptic properties, which can prevent and treat infections and help scars and burns heal faster. Because of this, rose water is often included in a variety of natural and medicinal treatments.

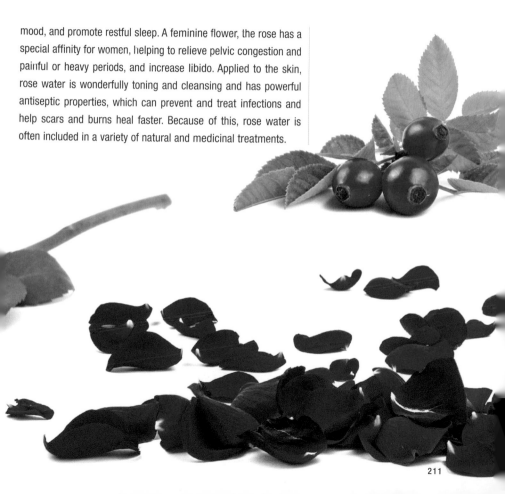

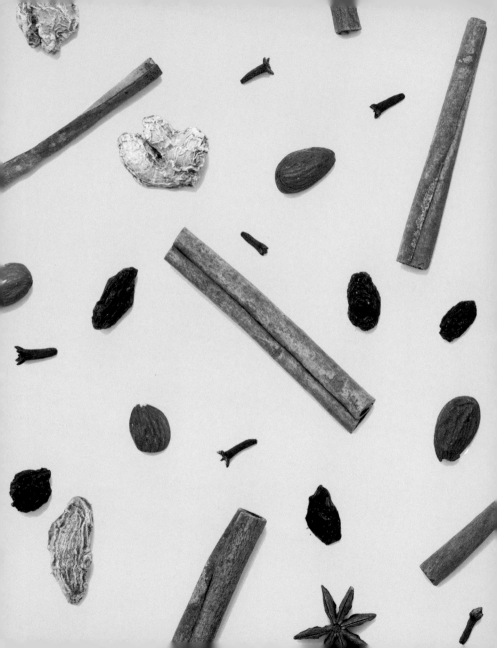

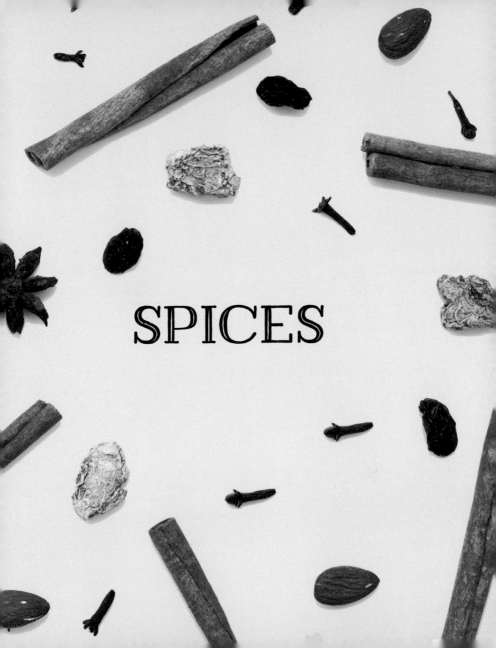

SPICES

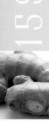

Ginger

PROPERTIES/ACTIONS
- Anti-nausea
- Carminitive
- Circulatory stimulant
- Boosts immunity
- Inhibits coughing

PARTS USED
- Root

Ginger is a favourite spice and flavouring, and one of the world's greatest medicines.

Used in India and China since 5000BCE, ginger is grown throughout the tropics and used extensively as both a culinary and therapeutic spice. It contains an active constituent, gingerol, which is responsible for much of its hot, pungent taste and aroma, as well as its stimulating properties. Ginger's volatile oil also lends many medicinal effects, working on the digestive system by encouraging secretion of digestive enzymes. Ginger is a wonderful remedy for indigestion, wind and colic. It invigorates the stomach and intestines, and relieves complaints such as motion and morning sickness. Moving stagnation of food and accumulation of toxins, including fungal infections, ginger increases vitality and enhances immunity.

GINGER & LEMON DECOCTION *for sore throats*

**115g (4oz) piece fresh ginger
zest and juice of 1 lemon
pinch of cayenne pepper**

Slice the ginger (there is no need to peel it) and put it in a saucepan together with the lemon zest, cayenne pepper and 500ml (17fl oz/ 2 cups) water. Bring to the boil,

cover the pan and simmer for 20 minutes. Remove from the heat and add the lemon juice. Drink 1 cup according to symptoms. The decoction will keep for 2–3 days.

Additionally, ginger is warming and soothing, and is a favourite home remedy for colds and influenza. It promotes perspiration, reducing a fever and clearing congestion, and has a stimulating and expectorant action in the lungs, expelling phlegm and relieving coughs. Ginger is also a useful remedy for pain and inflammation, helping cramps, peptic ulcers, allergies and asthma. It has a stimulating effect on the circulation, lowering high blood pressure.

The Roman Apicius included ginger in many recipes for sweet and savoury sauces.

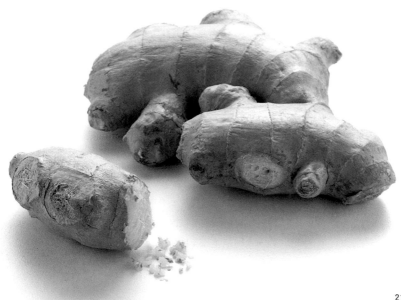

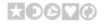

Turmeric

Grown for its root, turmeric is the most common flavour and colour present in Far Eastern cooking, and the root has a host of medicinal properties.

PROPERTIES/ACTIONS
- Treats liver
- Stimulates secretion of bile
- Analgesic
- Fights cancer
- Lowers cholesterol

PARTS USED
- Root

TURMERIC POULTICE
for skin inflammation

piece fresh turmeric root
gauze bandage

Grind the turmeric in a food processor to make a powder. Mix 1 tsp with a little water to make a paste. Wrap the paste in a bandage and tie to the affected area. Leave for 20 minutes, then discard. Repeat 3 times a day.

Turmeric is used in traditional Chinese medicine to treat the liver and gallbladder. It is a useful remedy that may help everything from gallstones and jaundice, to premenstrual discomfort and skin conditions. The spice is known to have effective anti-inflammatory and analgesic properties, good for treating arthritic and rheumatic problems as well as digestive disorders. Turmeric is high in antioxidants and due to its active ingredient, curcumin, has antibacterial and even cancer-fighting potential. It is an anti-coagulant, and has cholesterol-lowering properties.

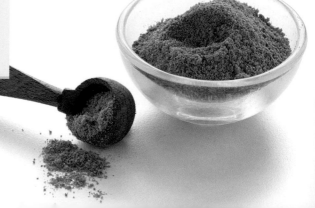

Cayenne Pepper

A fiery spice, cayenne pepper was first introduced to the West in the 16th century. It is a finely ground variety of chilli, with similar properties.

Cayenne, with the active constituent capsaicin, is a warming stimulant and a remedy for poor circulation. Applied to the skin, capsaicin desensitizes nerve endings and acts as a counter-irritant, helping local blood flow. It may help psoriasis, neuralgia, headaches and arthritis. Cayenne is taken to relieve wind and colic and to stimulate secretion of the digestive juices, as well as to aid metabolism.

The name "cayenne" derives from that of a French Guianan town of the same name.

PROPERTIES/ACTIONS
- Stimulant
- Improves circulation
- Treats wind & colic
- Aids metabolism

PARTS USED
- Fresh & dried pepper

CAYENNE-INFUSED OIL
for the skin

100g (3½oz/⅝ cup) finely chopped cayenne pepper
500ml (17fl oz/2 cups) vegetable or olive oil

Place the cayenne and oil in a heat-proof bowl. Bring a large saucepan of water to the boil, then reduce the heat and simmer gently. Set the bowl over the saucepan and leave for 2–3 hours. Remove from the heat and allow to cool. Strain the infused oil, using a funnel, into a dark glass bottle. Apply to the skin when needed.

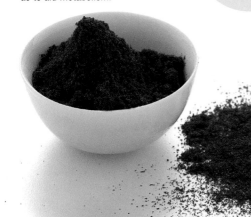

Anise

Used for centuries as a folk medicine as well as a spice, anise seed and its fruit, star anise, have similar therapeutic properties.

PROPERTIES/ACTIONS
- Stimulant
- Oestrogenic
- Relieves muscle spasm

PARTS USED
- Seed & fruit

HONEYED PEARS WITH ANISEED *for coughs*

½ tsp aniseed
1 pear, cored and sliced
1 dried fig
1 date
1 tsp honey

Place all the ingredients in a small saucepan. Cover and simmer gently for 45 minutes, or until the fruit is soft. Remove from the heat and eat immediately.

Anise seed is a good remedy to ease griping, intestinal colic and flatulence. It has marked expectorant action and may be used for bronchitis and for persistent, irritable coughing. With mild oestrogenic effects, anise seed can be used to increase milk secretion in lactating women. The fruit of the anise plant, known as star anise, has a similar effect, but with its ability to relieve muscle spasms, it is also used in herbal remedies for rheumatism, back pain and hernias. Star anise is also used for toothache. Both the seed and the fruit act as a heart stimulant.

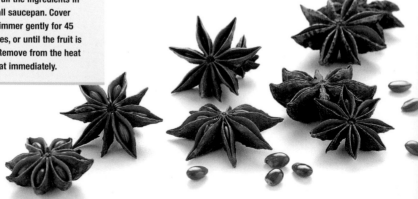

Nutmeg

Nutmeg has been an important part of the spice trade since the 6th century. It has also long been valued for its effect on the digestive system.

Nutmeg has a natural stimulating and anaesthetic effect on the stomach and intestines, and may help to reduce nausea and vomiting. It can also be a helpful remedy for gastroenteritis, and is excellent for treating diarrhoea, helping to warm the intestines and relieve abdominal pain.

In Ayurvedic medicine, nutmeg is a remedy for insomnia and coughs, and is believed to promote healthy skin. With a counter-irritant effect, it stimulates blood flow, helping to treat rheumatic conditions and eczema.

PROPERTIES/ACTIONS
- Stimulant
- Reduces nausea
- Helps diarrhoea
- Promotes healthy skin

PARTS USED
- Seed

SPICED NUTMEG SALVE
for rheumatism & inflammed skin

50g (2oz) petroleum jelly
1 tsp coarsley grated nutmeg
6 drops neroli essential oil

Melt the jelly in a bowl over a pan of simmering water. Stir in the nutmeg and leave for 30 minutes. Strain through a muslin (cheesecloth), leave to cool slightly, then add the essential oil. Pour into a glass jar and leave until set. Use as needed.

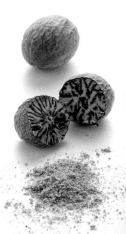
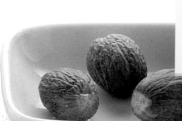

Black Cumin

Also known as nigella, black cumin is a traditional Asian remedy for gastro-intestinal disorders.

NUTRIENTS

Vitamins B1, B2; manganese, potassium; omega-3 and -6 fatty acids; volatile oils

---

SPICE TEA *serves 1*

1 tbsp black cumin seeds
1 tsp manuka honey
boiling water

Add the seeds and honey to a mug, then pour on enough boiling water to fill it, stirring continuously. Cover and leave for 10 minutes for the flavours to mingle, then drink.

Black cumin is a spice which has long been valued in Asia for its medicinal properties. Recent studies have suggested that it has powerful anti-microbial and anti-bacterial properties, and aids the recovery of the digestive system after food poisoning. Its essential fatty acids help to balance the immune system and to moderate allergic reactions, while its oil stimulates immune response, protecting against cancer. Black cumin also has an antimucosal effect, making it effective during colds and other infections of the respiratory tract.

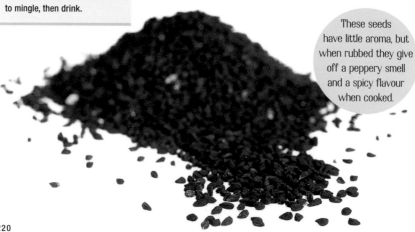

These seeds have little aroma, but when rubbed they give off a peppery smell and a spicy flavour when cooked.

Mustard Seed

NUTRIENTS
Vitamins B1, B2, B3, carotenoids; calcium, iron, magnesium, zinc; volatile oils

The Latin name *mustum ardens* **literally means "burning paste" – it's not hard to understand why!**

Mustard seed's potent volatile oils make it useful for helping to fight off colds. It stimulates the circulation and encourages sweating, helping to expel toxins. Mustard seed also contains small amounts of immunity-boosting minerals, including blood-enhancing iron and antioxidant zinc, as well as B-vitamins, which can increase energy.

MASALA CHICKEN

serves 4

2 tbsp ghee
2 onions, sliced
2 tsp grated fresh ginger
2 garlic cloves, crushed
1 red chilli, finely chopped
1 tsp black mustard seeds
2 tsp garam masala
2 tsp ground cumin
4 chicken breasts
125ml (4fl oz/½ cup) coconut milk
1 tbsp chopped coriander (cilantro)

Heat the ghee in a wok and stir-fry the onions, ginger and garlic for 2 minutes. Add the chilli and spices, and stir-fry for 3 minutes. Add the chicken and 250ml (9fl oz/1 cup) water and simmer until the chicken is tender. Add the coconut milk and coriander, and stir until heated through.

Mustard seed can be an irritant if used excessively, so always use it sparingly.

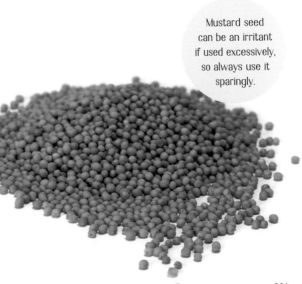

Cinnamon

This fragrant spice provides a satisfying alternative for people who find it difficult to resist unhealthy sugary snacks.

NUTRIENTS
Vitamins B2, B3, B5, B6, E, K, beta-carotene; calcium, copper, iodine, iron, magnesium, manganese, phosphorus, potassium, selenium, zinc

STABILIZES BLOOD SUGAR

Research has shown that compounds in cinnamon stabilize blood-sugar levels, which in turn prevent mood swings and dips in blood sugar post-exercise – a time when even the most health-conscious person might be tempted to succumb to calorie-laden chocolate and sweets. As little as half a teaspoonful a day – sprinkled on porridge for breakfast or used to sweeten a cup of herbal tea – can make a difference and, say scientists, even help to control type-2 diabetes.

CINNAMON FACTS

• Cinnamon is a spice made from the inner bark of the *Cinnamomum zeylanicum* tree. The bark is stripped from the tree and allowed to dry in the sun. While drying, it rolls up into a quill (sold as a cinnamon stick). Some of the quills are then ground into a powder.

• Cinnamon is one of the oldest-known spices. It was mentioned in ancient Chinese writings 2,700 years ago and features several times in the Bible.

• Ceylon cinnamon has a lighter, sweeter and more delicate flavour than the Indonesian variety.

APPLE AND CINNAMON PORRIDGE

2 cinnamon sticks
5 cloves
2 tsp sugar
2 apples, peeled
  and sliced
125g (4½oz/1¼ cups)
  instant porridge oats

In a large pan, bring 750ml (26fl oz/3 cups) of water to the boil. Reduce the heat, add the cinnamon, cloves, sugar and apple, and simmer for 10 minutes. Remove the spices, stir in the oats and serve.

PREVENTS THRUSH

Cinnamon also has anti-bacterial and anti-fungal properties that have been found to inhibit organisms such as *Candida albicans,* a yeast responsible for causing candidiasis and thrush.

CINNAMON TEA

4 heaped tsp black tea leaves
4 cinnamon sticks
1 lemon, sliced

Place the black tea, cinnamon sticks and lemon slices in a pan and pour over 1 litre (35fl oz/ 4 cups) freshly boiled water. Allow to steep for 5 minutes. Pour through a strainer into four cups and serve.

Cinnamon's distinct smell works directly on the brain to increase alertness.

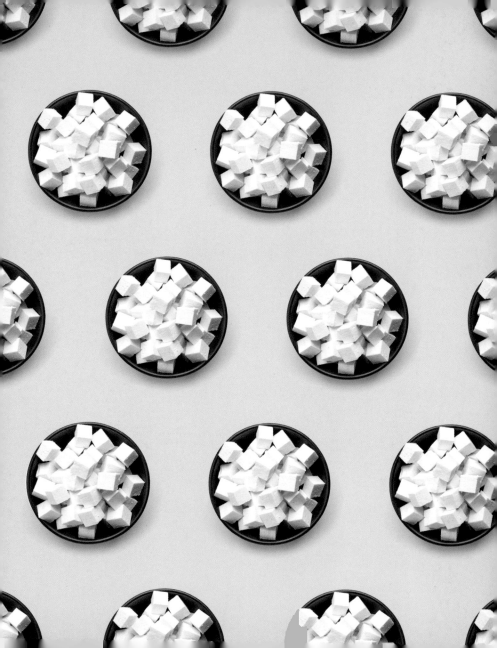

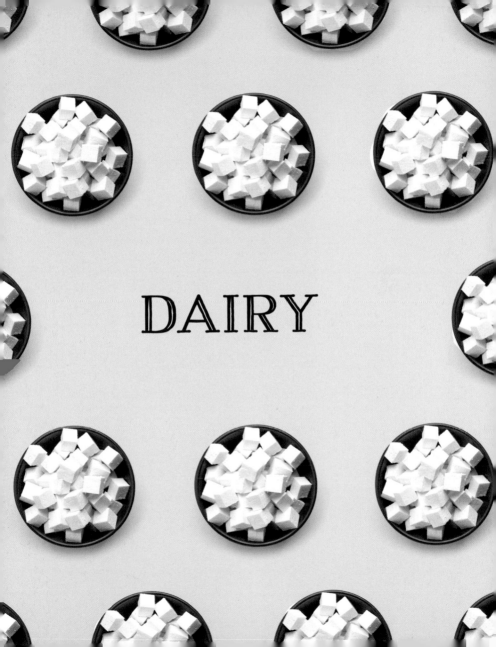

DAIRY

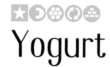

Yogurt

PROPERTIES/ACTIONS
- Contains "friendly" bacteria
- Fights infections
- Helps stomach ulcers
- Rich in calcium

PARTS USED
- Fermented milk

Ancient Bedouins discovered that heat and movement fermented the milk to create yogurt.

A cultured milk product, yogurt is positively brimming with "friendly" bacteria and many health-promoting nutrients.

Containing live cultures such as *Lactobacillus* and *Bifida* bacteria, yogurt stimulates the production of anti-viral and antibacterial agents and helps to fight off infections. These "friendly" bacteria attack and destroy the "bad" bacteria that cause food poisoning, as well as allowing the gut to absorb other essential nutrients efficiently.

The bacteria synthesize B vitamins, biotin, folic acid (folate) and vitamin B12, which helps fight depression, and increase the absorption of calcium and magnesium needed for healthy bones. Yogurt also supplies small traces of vitamin D, which is essential for the absorption of calcium.

YOGURT & EVENING PRIMROSE FACE MASK *for revitalizing & replenishing tired skin*

2 capsules evening primrose oil
2 capsules vitamin E oil
3 tbsp plain bio-yogurt
1 tsp honey
30g (1oz/¼ cup) potato flour

Extract the oil from the evening primrose and vitamin E oil capsules and combine it in a bowl with the other ingredients. Add extra flour to achieve the desired consistency.

Apply the mask evenly to the face and leave for approximately 20 minutes. Wash off with water and pat dry. Repeat the process each evening, as desired.

Yogurt is especially useful for preventing yeast infections that cause itching, burning and other uncomfortable symptoms, and offers some relief from stomach ulcers. It may also help to prevent cancer. Some studies have found that the probiotics present in yogurt produce enzymes that are absorbed directly through the gut wall, which further strengthens immune defences. Yogurt also provides an alternative for those who cannot tolerate the lactose in milk.

LASSI *South Indian yogurt drink*

250g (9oz/1 cup) plain yogurt
1 tsp cumin seeds
½ tsp salt
½ tsp finely chopped mint

Put all the ingredients in a blender with 625ml (21fl oz/ 2½ cups) water and whizz for a few seconds, until well mixed. Serve cold.

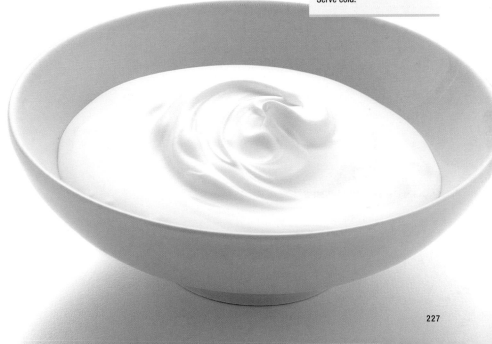

Cheese

NUTRIENTS
Vitamins A, B2, B12; calcium, iodine, phosphorus, selenium

Eating cheese tops up the body's levels of the crucial nutrients calcium and protein.

Weight-bearing exercise builds strong bones, but it puts them under pressure, increasing the body's need for calcium, which builds bone density. This means that cheese makes an ideal snack for athletes or sports players, who also lose calcium in perspiration. In fact, 30 minutes of sweat-inducing exercise increases calcium requirement. Cheese can get a bad press for its high saturated-fat content, but studies show that eating it after a meal actually boosts the body's ability to burn fat.

REALLY CHEESY SAUCE

55g (2oz/¼ cup) butter
2 tbsp plain (all-purpose) flour
400ml (14fl oz/1¾ cups)
  semi-skimmed milk
85g (3oz) Stilton, crumbled
55g (2oz/1¼ cups) grated
  Parmesan
½ tsp mustard
pinch of cayenne pepper
½ tsp grated nutmeg
wholemeal pasta, to serve

Melt the butter in a pan, add the flour and a little of the milk and stir to form a paste. Stirring over a gentle heat, add the rest of the milk. Bring to the boil, then remove from the heat. Add the Stilton and Parmesan, and stir in the mustard, cayenne pepper and nutmeg. Serve over wholemeal pasta.

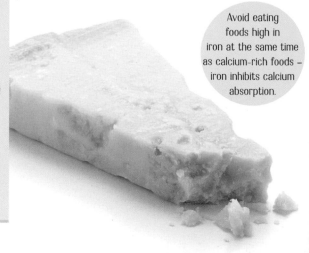

Avoid eating foods high in iron at the same time as calcium-rich foods – iron inhibits calcium absorption.

Milk

Milk is soothing and comforting, and provides liquid nutrition that is helpful in preventing and treating a great many conditions.

Milk is a first-class protein, providing building blocks that are especially useful in a child's diet. It is a rich source of calcium, which strengthens the bones and prevents osteoporosis, as well as some B vitamins, iron and zinc. Some studies show that milk may be good for the brain and for preventing strokes. It may contain substances that reduce the liver's production of cholesterol and lower blood pressure.

Irish folk medicine states that sheep droppings were given in milk for whooping cough.

PROPERTIES/ACTIONS
- First-class protein
- Rich in calcium
- Strengthens bones

PARTS USED
- Milk

MILK & HONEY BATH LOTION *to nourish the skin*

2 eggs
3 tbsp carrier oil
150ml (5fl oz/⅔ cup) milk
2 tsp honey
2 tsp organic shampoo
1 tbsp vodka

In a bowl, beat together the eggs and oil. Add the other ingredients, mix and pour into a glass bottle. Add 30–45ml (1–1½fl oz/2–3 tbsp) to bath water. Keep the remaining lotion chilled and use within 3–4 days.

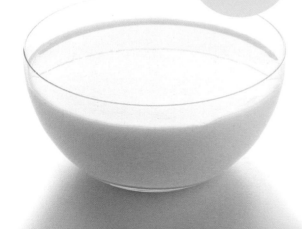

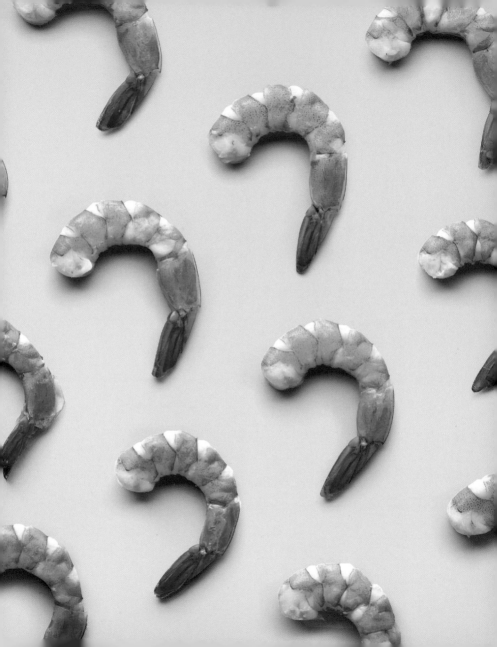

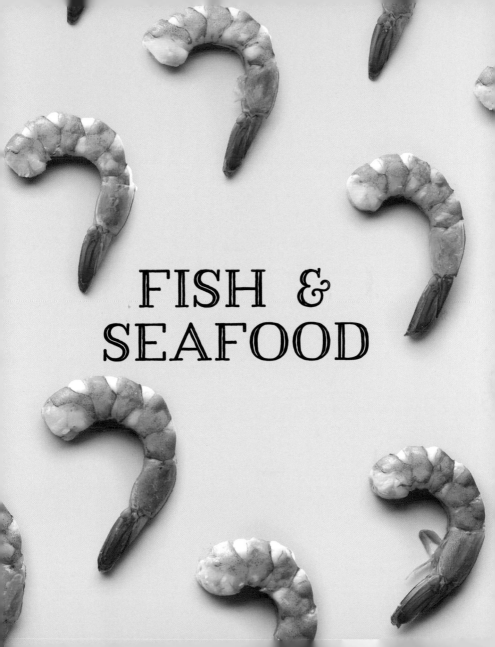

FISH & SEAFOOD

◐▶◭♥◉⊕

Salmon

Containing a wealth of omega-3 fatty acids and other health-giving properties, salmon is essential to the diet.

The deeper the colour of salmon, the more beneficial omega-3 fatty acids it contains.

PROPERTIES/ACTIONS
- Rich in omega-3 fatty acids
- Good for skin
- Promotes healthy nervous system
- Treats behavioural problems

PARTS USED
- Salmon

Salmon is a source of protein, minerals and B vitamins. Being high in omega-3 it regulates immune-boosting white blood cells, prevents high blood pressure, lowers blood cholesterol, may help conditions of the central nervous system, reduces inflammation and could even help fight against cancer. It is especially good for arthritis and skin conditions such as psoriasis and eczema.

SIZZLING SALMON *serves 4*

500g (1lb 2oz) salmon fillet
½ tsp dried chilli/hot pepper flakes
¼ tsp paprika
4 tsp olive oil
sea salt and black pepper
4 tsp chopped coriander (cilantro), to serve

Cut the salmon into four. Place skin-side down on a griddle pan and sprinkle with the chilli, paprika and oil. Season with salt and pepper, and cook for 6–8 minutes. Place the salmon on four serving plates and sprinkle with the chopped coriander. Serve immediately.

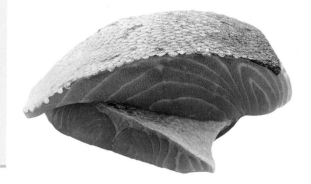

Fresh Tuna

A member of the mackerel family, tuna is rich in healthy oils and immunity-boosting minerals.

NUTRIENTS
Vitamins B3, B6, B12, D, E; iodine, selenium; omega-3 fatty acids

Tuna contains vitamin E and selenium, which are needed for the production of disease-fighting antibodies, and many B-vitamins, which enhance energy. Like other oily fish, it has high levels of omega-3 fatty acids, a family of essential fatty acids that can help to prevent heart disease, cancer and depression. Omega-3s also play a role in balancing the immune system, helping to reduce allergic reactions. They are also anti-inflammatory, calming conditions such as rheumatoid arthritis and eczema.

Always choose fresh rather than canned tuna, as the canning process destroys omega 3 fats.

TUNA NIÇOISE *serves 4*

juice of 1 lemon
½ tsp salt
1 tsp Dijon mustard
5 tbsp olive oil
pinch of black pepper
4 tuna steaks
4 medium potatoes, cooked and sliced

115g (4oz) green beans
115g (4oz) mixed salad leaves
4 tomatoes, cut into segments
handful of black olives

Whisk together the lemon juice, salt, mustard, olive oil and black pepper. Place the tuna steaks on a large plate and coat in the dressing mixture. Chill for 1 hour, then grill (broil) for 4–6 minutes. Combine all the vegetables in a large salad bowl and drizzle over the remaining dressing. Top with the tuna steaks and serve.

Trout

NUTRIENTS

Vitamins A, B1, B2, B6, B12; calcium, iron, selenium; omega-3 essential fatty acids

With a third of the fat of salmon, trout is an excellent alternative for the calorie-conscious.

Trout is a good source of essential fatty acids, which have been found to help increase an athlete's speed, because they improve the delivery of oxygen to the body's cells, boosting energy levels and building stamina. Omega-3 fats have also been found to stimulate production of a hormone called leptin, which helps to control appetite. In addition, trout is packed with protein to encourage muscle growth and repair.

One 100g/3½oz portion of trout contains just 135 calories.

TROUT STUFFED WITH SAGE AND ROSEMARY

serves 4

**4 fresh whole trout,
    gutted and cleaned
handful of sage
handful of rosemary
juice of 2 lemons
55g (2oz/¼ cup) butter
steamed greens, to serve**

Place the trout in an ovenproof dish. Stuff some herbs into each fish and drizzle with lemon juice. Melt the butter and pour over the fish. Bake in a pre-heated oven at 180°C/350°F/Gas 4 for 35 minutes. Serve with steamed greens.

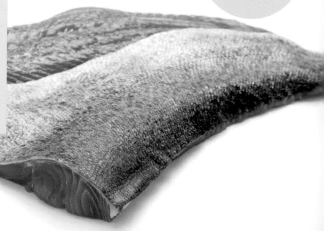

Sardine

Sardines are one of the few non-dairy sources of easily absorbable calcium.

NUTRIENTS

Vitamins B3, B6, D, E; calcium, iodine, iron, potassium, selenium; omega-3 essential fatty acids

JAPANESE SARDINES

serves 4

450g (1lb) sardines,
  washed and dried
125ml (4fl oz/½ cup) soy sauce
4 tbsp white wine vinegar
juice and zest of 1 lime
1 lemongrass stem,
  chopped
2.5cm (1in) piece root ginger,
  peeled and chopped
2 garlic cloves, crushed
1 tsp chilli powder

Arrange the sardines in a shallow dish. Mix together the remaining ingredients in a bowl and pour over the sardines. Cover and refrigerate for 3 hours. Discard the marinade and grill (broil) the sardines for 3–5 minutes, turning once, until the flesh flakes.

Including plenty of calcium in the diet is essential for strong bones and, according to research, can also help the body to burn body fat more efficiently. Sardines are packed with protein, iron, zinc, essential fatty acids and vitamin D, and are exceptionally rich in calcium. Ask the fishmonger to remove the heads and backbones, but leave the other bones – once cooked they're very soft and you can just mash them with a fork.

Canned sardines are an inexpensive, highly nutritious "instant" food.

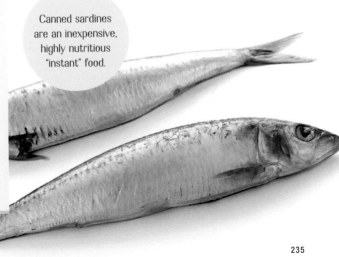

235

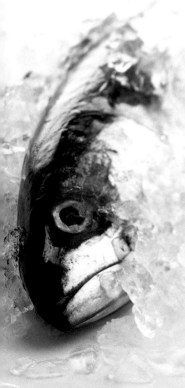

NUTRIENTS

Vitamins B3, B6, B12, D; iodine, potassium, selenium; omega-3 fatty acids

Mackerel

One of the best fish choices for overall health, mackerel is packed with nutrients.

Mackerel is an excellent source of omega-3 fatty acids, which help to keep cholesterol levels low and, studies suggest, could also be effective in preventing cancer and depression. Omega-3 fats are also important for healthy joints and skin. Mackerel contains vitamin B6, which the body needs in order to make key amino acids for immune health, and it is one of the few food sources of vitamin D, which is crucial for good bone development. In addition, mackerel is rich in selenium, an antioxidant mineral which is vital for immune function.

One serving a week of an oily fish, such as mackerel, can help to prevent heart disease.

SEARED MACKEREL AND FENNEL SALAD *serves 4*

2 bulbs fennel, sliced
1 tbsp olive oil
4 garlic cloves
4 oranges, peeled and sliced
4 fresh mackerel, filleted

Preheat the oven to 200°C/ 400°F/Gas 6. Place the fennel and garlic on a baking tray,

drizzle with olive oil and roast for 15 minutes. Add the orange slices and roast for a further 5 minutes. In a frying pan, fry the mackerel in the remaining olive oil for 5 minutes. Add the roasted ingredients, toss together for 2 minutes, then serve.

Fresh Anchovy

This small, slender oily fish is a good source of protein and omega-3 fatty acids.

Fresh anchovy is rich in omega-3 fatty acids, which the body converts to prostaglandins, substances essential for immune function, reducing inflammation, controlling levels of cholesterol and boosting mood. It is one of the best sources of vitamin D, which we need to moderate the immune system by reducing its activity when necessary, and is also vital for healthy bones. Anchovy also contains protein and B-vitamins – both needed for energy production.

NUTRIENTS
Vitamins B2, B3, D; calcium, iron, phosphorous; omega-3 fatty acids; protein

Anchovy is rich in iron, which is crucial for healthy blood and circulation.

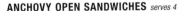

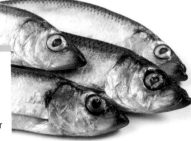

ANCHOVY OPEN SANDWICHES *serves 4*

4 slices rye bread
1 garlic clove, crushed
2 tbsp olive oil
100g (3½oz) cherry tomatoes,
    sliced
55g (2oz) canned anchovy
    fillets in olive oil, drained
sea salt and black pepper

Lightly toast the rye bread on both sides. Meanwhile, mix the garlic into the olive oil in a cup, and brush the mixture over the toast, when ready. Top with the tomatoes and anchovies, season and serve.

176

Crayfish

NUTRIENTS
Vitamins B3, B12; calcium, copper, magnesium, potassium, selenium, sulphur, zinc

Freshwater crustaceans, crayfish are loaded with immunity-boosting minerals.

Crayfish look like miniature versions of lobsters, to which they are closely related. They are an excellent source of selenium, an antioxidant mineral that research shows is one of the best natural cell-protectors around, as it mops up the free radicals produced by the body during exercise. A selenium deficiency is associated with anxiety, depression and fatigue. Crayfish is also a valuable source of zinc, which helps to ward off disease.

CRAYFISH TAGLIATELLE

300g (10½oz) fresh tagliatelle
500g (1lb 2oz) cherry tomatoes, halved
1 tbsp olive oil
juice and zest of 1 lemon
400g (14oz) cooked crayfish tails
handful of basil leaves

Cook the tagliatelle in a large pan of salted, boiling water for 6–8 minutes or as instructed on the package, then drain. In another pan, sauté the tomatoes in the oil for 3 minutes. Add the lemon juice and zest, crayfish, basil and tagliatelle, and serve.

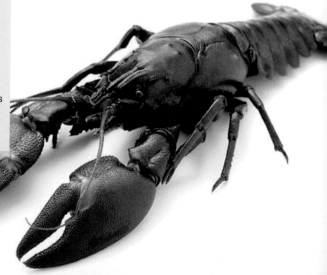

Prawn

The world's most popular crustaceans, prawns (shrimp) are rich in immunity-boosting nutrients.

Prawns contain high levels of immune-essential minerals, including zinc, which we need to produce the enzymes that keep cancer at bay, and to help develop other disease-fighting cells. These shellfish also contain selenium, a potent antioxidant mineral which helps in the production of antibodies, and improves the efficiency of white blood cells at recognising unwanted invaders. Prawns are a good source of protein, which is necessary for building healthy tissues and boosting energy.

NUTRIENTS
Vitamins B3, B12; calcium, iodine, magnesium, phosphorous, potassium, selenium, zinc; protein

PRAWNS WITH PEPPER SAUCE *serves 4*

4 red (bell) peppers, deseeded and chopped
1 tomato, chopped
2 garlic cloves, crushed
2 tbsp chopped parsley
1 tbsp white wine vinegar
800g (1lb 12oz) cooked prawns (shrimp)
1 Iceberg lettuce

Preheat the oven to 190°C/ 375°F/Gas 5 and place the peppers on a baking tray. Bake for 15 minutes until soft. Mix together in a bowl with the tomato, garlic, parsley and vinegar. Shred the lettuce and divide among four bowls. Peel the prawns and place a few in each bowl, before topping with the pepper mixture.

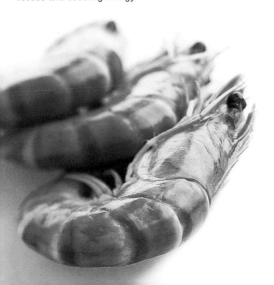

178

Oyster

PROPERTIES/ACTIONS
- High in iodine
- Enhances the reproductive system
- Rich in zinc
- High in vitamin E & omega-3 fats

PARTS USED
- Oyster

Oysters are bisexual, or inter-sexual, changing from males to females.

Oysters are a type of shellfish that is not only a renowned aphrodisiac, but also full of health-promoting vitamins, minerals and other nutrients.

Oysters are an excellent source of protein. They are rich in vitamin E and omega-3 fatty acids for heart health, and have many brain-boosting B vitamins, including B12, which helps fight fatigue. They also contain vitamin D, which is needed for healthy bones and teeth, as well as potassium, iron and selenium. In Chinese medicine, they supplement the liver and kidneys, and treat insomnia, restlessness and agitation.

Oysters have a well-documented affinity with the reproductive system. They are a rich source of iodine, which is necessary for the

OYSTERS AU PARMESAN

125g (4½oz/1 cup) breadcrumbs
1 tbsp butter
3 dozen fresh oysters
sea salt and cayenne pepper
15g (½oz/½ cup) chopped parsley
125g (4½oz/2 cups) grated Parmesan cheese
125ml (4fl oz/½ cup) white wine

Preheat the oven to 180°C/350°F/Gas 4. In a pan, brown the breadcrumbs in the butter, reserving 1 tbsp. Grease a shallow baking dish, then dust with the fried breadcrumbs. Season the oysters with salt and cayenne pepper and place them on top of the

breadcrumbs. Scatter the parsley and Parmesan cheese on top, followed by the remaining breadcrumbs. Pour the wine over the entire dish. Bake in the oven for 15 minutes. Serve hot.

proper functioning of the thyroid and the reproductive hormones. Research also indicates that certain sterols are present in oysters, from which the sex hormones are derived. They are used regularly by Chinese women to increase oestrogen in the body, and are useful for infertility and for treating menopausal disorders. Oysters are a rich natural source of nutrients, including zinc – just six raw oysters provide excellent amounts of this important nutrient. Zinc is essential for the production of sperm and enhances libido. It also helps to boost immunity.

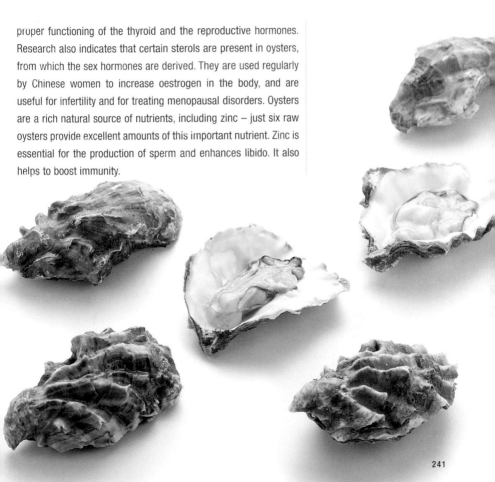

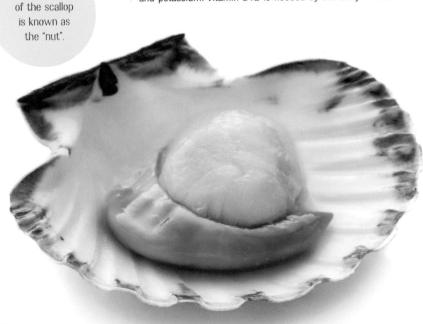

Scallop

NUTRIENTS
Vitamin B12; calcium, magnesium, phosphorus, potassium, selenium; omega-3 essential fatty acids

A type of mollusc with a soft, fleshy texture and a delicate, mild flavour, scallops are loaded with heart-friendly nutrients.

Scallops provide four nutrients that have significant cardio-vascular benefits – vitamin B12, omega-3 essential fatty acids, magnesium and potassium. Vitamin B12 is needed by the body to counteract

The edible part of the scallop is known as the "nut".

homocysteine, a chemical that can directly damage blood vessel walls; omega-3 fats help the blood to flow smoothly; magnesium encourages blood vessels to relax, lowering blood pressure; and potassium aids in the maintenance of normal blood pressure levels. Studies have proven that scallops are able to reduce the risk of stroke by as much as 31 per cent. The essential minerals and rich dose of antioxidants reduces dangerous clotting, improves circulation and keeps your brain full of healthy blood.

GRILLED CORIANDER SCALLOPS

24 scallops, shelled and
   shells reserved
115g (4oz/½ cup) butter
juice of ½ lime
small handful of coriander
   (cilantro) leaves, chopped

Place the scallops flesh side up on a baking tray. Cook under a hot grill (broiler) for 2 minutes. Divide the butter, lime juice and coriander between the shells. Cook for another 2–3 minutes until the scallops are white all the way through, and serve.

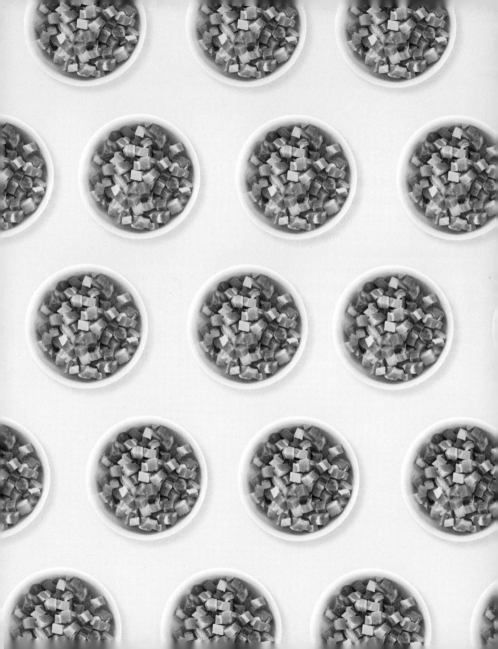

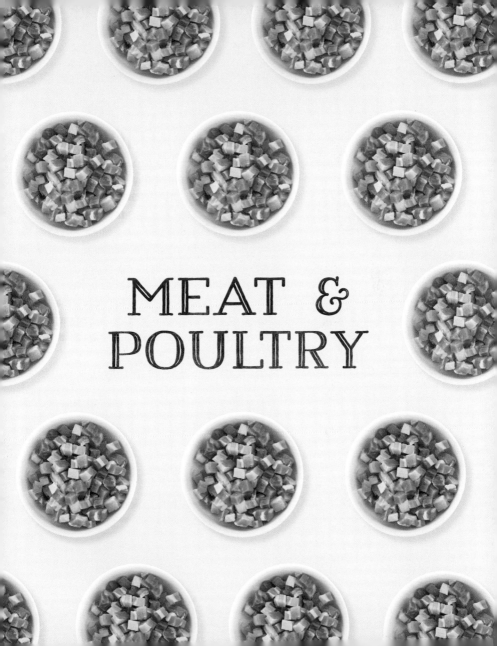

MEAT & POULTRY

Lamb

As well as being a traditional symbol of continuing life and resurrection, lamb has valuable nutritional properties.

PROPERTIES/ACTIONS
- Rich in protein
- Prevents anaemia
- Boosts immunity
- Improves circulation

PARTS USED
- Lamb

Like other red meat, lamb is rich in protein, as well as being an excellent source of two vital minerals: iron and zinc. Iron helps to boost the oxygen-carrying capability of blood, preventing anaemia and fatigue from setting in, while zinc is necessary for optimum functioning of the immune system, helping to fight colds, infections and other invaders.

According to the Chinese, eating lamb improves circulation, overcomes coldness, and may even treat post-natal depression.

LAMB KOFTA *serves 4*

450g (1lb) minced (ground) lamb
1 large onion, grated
1 tsp salt
30g (1oz/1 cup) finely chopped parsley
¼ tsp black pepper
1 tsp ground allspice

Combine the ingredients and chill for 1 hour. Divide and shape into balls, then thread the balls onto skewers. Cook under the grill (broiler) until browned on all sides and cooked through.

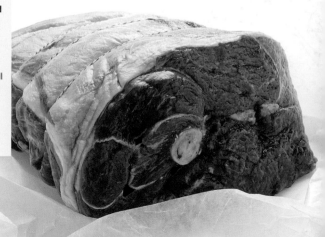

Beef

Reserved in Britain for the ruling Normans until after the 13th century, beef is a flavourful meat with many therapeutic attributes.

A rich source of animal protein, beef has high levels of iron, zinc and many B-complex vitamins, and may help to protect against chronic fatigue syndrome, anaemia, weak digestion, depression and mood swings. According to the Chinese eating beef lifts body metabolism, treats hypoglycaemia and strengthens bones. Organic beef is free from pesticides and contains conjugated linoleic acid, which has cancer-fighting properties and stimulates the conversion of stored fat into energy.

PROPERTIES/ACTIONS
- Rich in iron, zinc & B vitamins
- Prevents anaemia
- Good for mood swings

PARTS USED
- Beef

PEPPER STEAKS *serves 4*

4 beef fillet steaks
2 tbsp olive oil
6 tbsp assorted cracked peppercorns
2 garlic cloves, crushed
40g (1½oz/2½ tbsp) butter
sea salt

Coat the steaks with the olive oil. Press down on the peppercorns, then press them into the steaks. Coat the steaks thoroughly with the crushed garlic. Melt the butter in a large frying pan. Cook the steaks over a medium heat for 3–4 minutes on each side. Season to taste with salt.

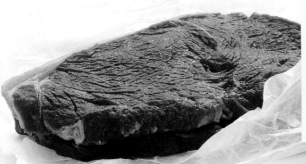

NATURE'S PHARMACY

Pork

NUTRIENTS
Vitamins B1, B2, B3, B6, B12;
potassium, selenium, zinc

Pork is a valuable source of two trusty energy providers – protein and the B-vitamin complex.

While eating in general raises the metabolic rate, protein boosts it the most: up to 20 per cent of a protein meal's calories may be burned off. An average portion of pork (100g/3½oz) contains 30g/1oz of pure protein. It also has a full house of B-vitamins, which are essential for converting carbohydrates into energy and preventing fatigue.

ROAST GAMMON WITH PLUM GLAZE *serves 8*

125g (4½oz) plum jam
juice and zest of 1 orange
1 tsp ground nutmeg
1 tsp ground cinnamon
1 tsp ground ginger
2.25kg (5lb) unsmoked
gammon joint

Place the jam, orange and spices in a small pan, gently heat together and brush the mixture over the joint. Wrap joint in foil and roast in a pre-heated oven at 190°C/375°F/Gas 5 for 2½ hours. Remove the foil and roast for a further 30 minutes. Carve and serve.

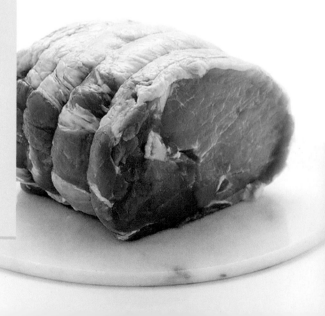

Turkey

Often reserved for festive occasions, nutritious turkey can be an everyday health-booster.

An excellent low-fat source of protein, turkey is rich in immunity-fortifying zinc, in a form that is easy for the body to use. It also contains selenium, which helps to repair cell DNA and lower the risk of cancer. Turkey is dense in B-vitamins, which are needed for a healthy nervous system and are important for keeping down levels of homocysteine in the blood. This is a toxic substance formed as a breakdown product of amino acids and linked with heart disease.

NUTRIENTS
Vitamins B3, B6, B12; iron, selenium, zinc; protein

DELUXE TURKEY SANDWICH *serves 1*

½ avocado
2 slices wholegrain bread
fresh spinach leaves
cooked turkey slices
1 spring onion (scallion), finely
  chopped
1 tomato, sliced
a little wholegrain mustard

Scoop out the avocado flesh and spread over the bread like butter. Layer the spinach and turkey slices on one slice and top with the onion, tomato, and mustard. Sandwich together and eat immediately.

Dark turkey leg meat contains twice as much iron and three times as much zinc as white breast meat.

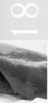

Chicken

NUTRIENTS

Vitamins A, B2, B3, B6, B12, K; iron, magnesium, phosphorus, potassium, selenium, sodium, zinc

CHICKEN FACTS

• A chicken breast with the skin on contains almost twice as much saturated fat as a skinned chicken breast.

• The white breast meat of chicken contains less fat and fewer calories than the dark meat (wings and legs).

• Free-range poultry doesn't contain any of the growth-promoting hormones or antibiotics given to intensively reared birds.

• Chicken is cooked when it's opaque and there's no trace of pink at the bone, and the juices run clear.

Rated as a protein powerhouse, chicken is perhaps the most versatile meat of all.

A high intake of saturated fats increases the risk of heart disease and piles on the kilos/pounds. While all meat and dairy products contain some saturated fat, chicken, particularly if organic, is one of the leanest, most health-enhancing choices.

ENHANCES PERFORMANCE

Chicken provides a good deal of protein to build and repair muscles and an impressive list of minerals, including magnesium to help reduce the risk of cramps during exercise, and potassium to

---

BALSAMIC CHICKEN DRUMSTICKS *serves 4*

6 tbsp balsamic vinegar
2 tbsp sunflower oil
1 tsp Dijon mustard
1 tsp clear honey
½ tsp salt
1 tsp black pepper
8 large chicken drumsticks

In a bowl, mix the vinegar, oil, mustard and honey, and season. Coat the drumsticks, and chill in a shallow dish for 2 hours. Grill (broil) for 15–20 minutes, turning every 5 minutes until cooked through and the juices run clear, then serve.

balance the fluid levels in the body, as well as selenium and zinc to bolster immunity. Zinc is also known to have energy-boosting properties.

LIFTS MOOD

Chicken is an excellent source of tryptophan, an essential amino acid that helps to control the brain's serotonin levels, which are linked to appetite and mood. The B-complex vitamins also help to regulate the metabolism.

A 1–1.35kg (2–3lb) chicken can be frozen whole for eight months and will take 10–12 hours to thaw.

THAI CHICKEN serves 4

1 tsp chilli powder
2.5cm (1in) piece root ginger, peeled and grated
juice and zest of 1 lime
4 boneless chicken breasts, cut into strips
400ml (14fl oz/1¾ cups) coconut milk
400ml (14fl oz/1¾ cups) chicken stock

In a bowl, mix the chilli powder, ginger, and lime juice and zest. Place the chicken in a dish, pour over the marinade, cover and chill for 1 hour. Bring the milk and stock to the boil in a pan. Add the chicken and simmer for 15 minutes.

Guinea Fowl

NUTRIENTS
Vitamins B3, B6, B12; iron; protein

This protein-rich meat is high in nutrients.

Choose organic guinea fowl, as conventional birds are farmed intensively and can be low in nutrients.

A small game bird thought to have originated in West Africa, guinea fowl is a healthy, low-fat source of protein. It contains good levels of vitamin B6, which is needed for the synthesis of cysteine, an important amino acid, and also to help eliminate waste matter from the body. As with all meat, guinea fowl contains vitamin B12, which helps maintain an efficient nervous system, and iron, which we need for healthy blood.

HERBY GUINEA FOWL *serves 2*

1 tbsp chopped parsley
1 tbsp chopped tarragon
2 guinea fowl breasts
2 tsp olive oil
sea salt and black pepper

Preheat the oven to 200°C/
400°F/Gas 6. Stuff the chopped

herbs under the skin of the guinea fowl, and season as required. In a pan, heat the olive oil, and fry the breasts for 2 minutes on each side to brown, then transfer to the oven and cook for a further 8 minutes.

Pheasant

Rich in B vitamins and protein, pheasant is a good source of energy.

Pheasant is by far the most plentiful and popular of game birds. It is higher in fat than many other meats but the main fat it contains is the health-enhancing monounsaturated type, which is a plus. It also contains good levels of nutrients, so it is very beneficial when eaten occasionally. It is a useful source of vitamin B6, which is needed for the production of phagocytes to keep the body's cells healthy, and vitamins B2, B3 and B12 – vital for maintaining a healthy nervous system and consistent energy levels. It is also an excellent source of the immunity-boosting minerals, iron and zinc. However, pheasant is high in purines so should be avoided by those prone to gout.

NUTRIENTS
Vitamins B2, B3, B6, B12; iron, potassium, zinc; protein

PHEASANT STIR-FRY
serves 2

2 pheasant breast halves, skinned
2 tbsp sesame oil
1 onion, finely chopped
1 red (bell) pepper, deseeded and chopped
10 portobello mushrooms, sliced
2 tsp tamari soy sauce
brown rice or noodles, to serve

Cut the pheasant portions into large pieces, then fry on a low heat in the oil until browned. Add the onion, pepper and mushrooms and stir-fry together for around 6 minutes until the vegetables are tender and the pheasant cooked through. Add the soy sauce and serve with brown rice or noodles.

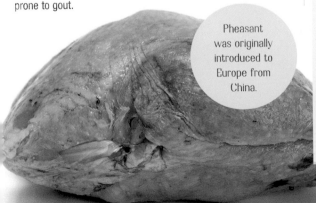

Pheasant was originally introduced to Europe from China.

187

Duck

NUTRIENTS
Vitamin B2; iron, zinc; protein

Duck is delicious roasted or stir-fried and is an excellent source of the stress-busting vitamin B2.

Duck is a popular and uniquely tasty variety of poultry and is a wonderful source of immune-boosting nutrients. Although duck is high in cholesterol, it is low in saturated fat. A skinless duck breast is leaner than a skinless chicken breast. Duck meat provides plenty of the protein and iron needed to repair tissue and build new cells. Eating duck will also help you to combat stress as it contains the vitamin B2 and aids the production of infection-fighting immune cells.

Ducks were first domesticated in China, where they are appreciated for their eggs.

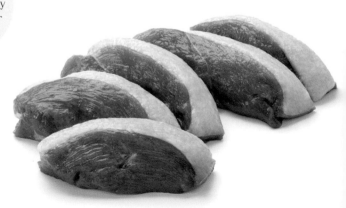

GLAZED DUCK WITH HONEY AND MUSTARD *serves 2*

1 tbsp runny honey
1 tbsp wholegrain mustard
2 duck breasts, skinned
oil, for roasting and frying
2 heads pak choi (bok choy),
  trimmed and ribboned
110g (4oz) brown rice, cooked

Preheat the oven to 190°C/ 375°F/ Gas 5. Mix the honey and mustard in a small bowl to form a marinade. Coat the duck breasts with the marinade and then place them in a lightly oiled roasting pan. Pour over any remaining marinade. Cover and bake for 20 minutes or until cooked through. While the duck is cooking, stir-fry the pak choi in a little oil. When the duck is ready, leave it to sit for a few minutes before serving with the freshly cooked rice and pak choi.

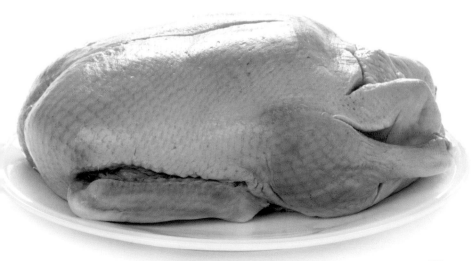

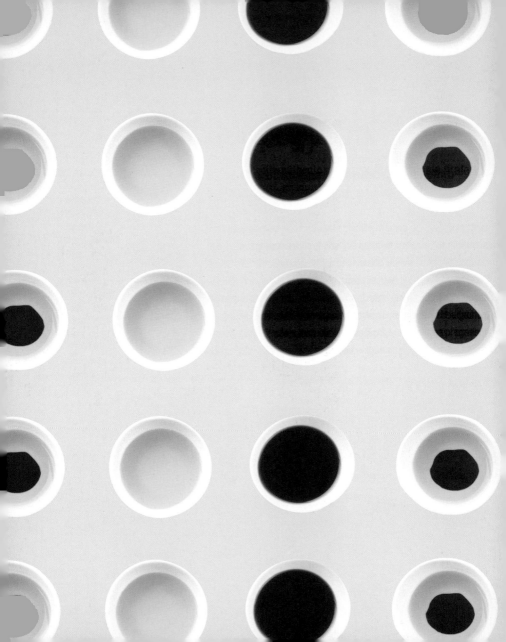

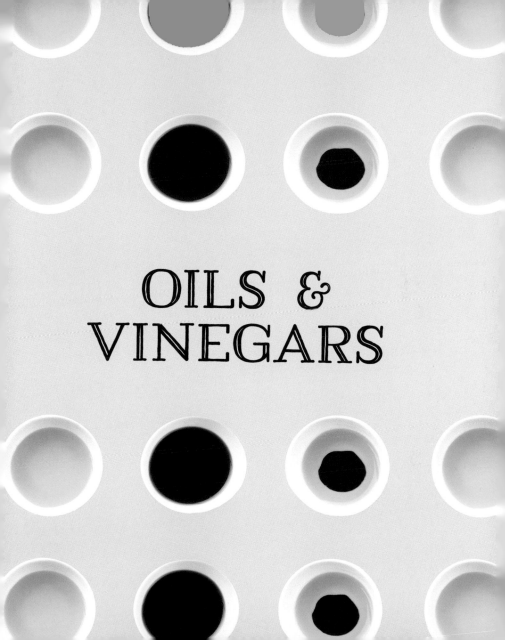

OILS & VINEGARS

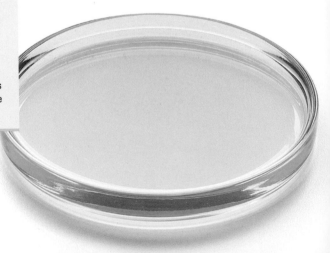

Cider Vinegar

Made from fermented apple juice and rich in enzymes, cider vinegar has been used for centuries to aid digestion.

Apart from its beneficial action on the digestion, cider vinegar helps symptoms such as heartburn and improves metabolism. The enzymes also help to dissolve calcium deposits, making it a popular joint health aid. Cider vinegar contains cholesterol-supporting pectin, which is good for heart health, and the perfect balance of 19 minerals. It has many system-cleansing benefits, while topically it maintains healthy skin.

PROPERTIES/ACTIONS
- Aids digestion
- Rich in enzymes
- Good for arthritis
- Contains pectin
- Promotes healthy skin

PARTS USED
- Cider vinegar

OXYMEL (TRADITIONAL MEDICINAL DRINK)

apple cider vinegar
pure honey

Combine equal amounts of apple cider vinegar and honey in a glass jar. Shake to combine. Take 1 tsp with symptoms, or add eight times the amount of water to create a juice for regular sipping.

Olive Oil

Central to the Mediterranean diet, olive oil appears to lower the risk of heart disease, as well as treating many other complaints.

Olive oil is a monounsaturated fat that lowers levels of harmful LDL cholesterol while leaving the beneficial HDL cholesterol alone. It contains other heart-healthy compounds, as well as antioxidants. Rich in vitamin E, it also stimulates the secretion of bile, helping to soften and expel gallstones.

Olive oil was used for anointing the body in ancient Greek religious rituals.

PROPERTIES/ACTIONS
- Lowers LDL cholesterol
- Rich in vitamin E
- Stimulates secretion of bile
- Laxative

PARTS USED
- Whole ripe olives

CAPER & OLIVE OIL TAPENADE *serves 4*

125ml (4fl oz/½ cup) extra virgin olive oil
5 tbsp capers
80g (2¾oz/½ cup) pitted green olives
2 anchovy fillets
4 garlic cloves

Blend the ingredients in a food processor. Serve with bread.

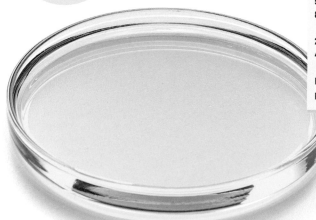

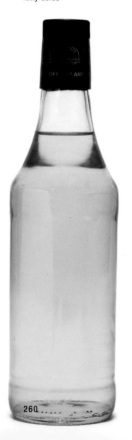

Safflower Oil

This light, golden oil from safflower seeds helps to prevent heart disease.

NUTRIENTS
Vitamin E; phytosterols; omega-6 fatty acids

Safflower oil is dense in vitamin E, an antioxidant which helps to ward off cancer, keep skin healthy, and detoxify the body. It also contains phytosterols, plant chemicals that can help to lower cholesterol and therefore help prevent heart disease and strokes. Safflower oil is rich in omega-6 fatty acids, which the body converts into prostaglandins that balance the immune system and stop allergic reactions, as well as thin the blood, soothe inflammation, improve nerve and brain function and aid the regulation of blood sugar levels. It is a polyunsaturate so it should not be heated and cold-pressed varieties always used.

SAFFLOWER VINAIGRETTE *makes 1 small bowl*

50ml (1¾fl oz/3½ tbsp) white wine vinegar
2 tsp Dijon mustard
150ml (5fl oz/⅔ cup) safflower oil
sea salt and black pepper

Whisk the vinegar and mustard together in a bowl and season with salt and pepper. Slowly drizzle in the oil, whisking until the ingredients are thoroughly combined. Use immediately, or store in a jar. Shake well before use.

Evening Primrose Oil

This healing flower oil stabilises hormones and boosts skin health.

Evening primrose oil is one of the richest known direct sources of gamma linoleic acid (GLA), an omega-6 fatty acid. In the body, this substance is converted into prostaglandins, hormone-like substances which help to regulate the immune system, thin the blood, decrease inflammation and improve nerve and muscle function. Increasing the body's levels of prostaglandins may also ease PMS symptoms. In addition, evening primrose oil is rich in vitamin E, which can help to boost skin health and ease conditions such as eczema.

NUTRIENTS
Vitamin E; gamma linoleic acid; omega-6 fatty acids

EVENING PRIMROSE SALAD DRESSING *makes 1 small bowl*

1 tbsp balsamic vinegar
3 tbsp lemon juice
1 tsp wholegrain mustard
1 tbsp parsley
1 tbsp chopped chives
1 garlic clove, chopped
1 tsp dried oregano
1 tsp dried basil
3 tbsp evening primrose oil

pinch of cayenne pepper
sea salt

In a blender, combine the vinegar, mustard, herbs and garlic. Blend until smooth. Slowly add the oil, then blend again until creamy. Season with cayenne and salt.

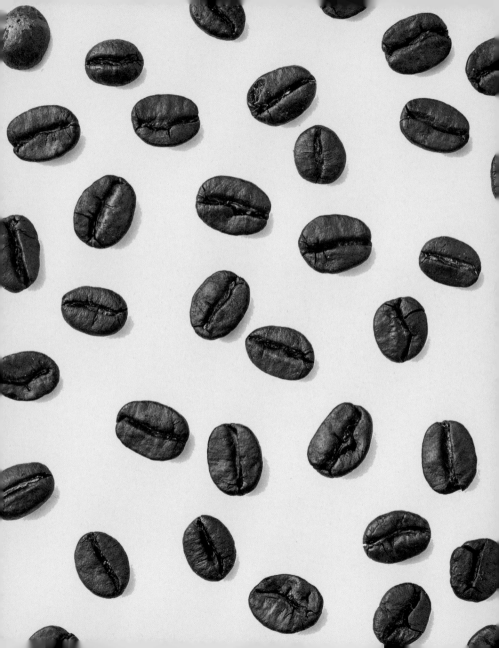

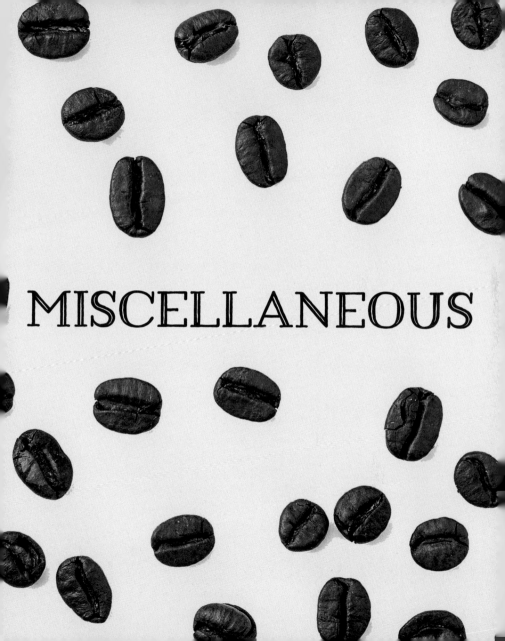

MISCELLANEOUS

192

⊗★▷◉◎◌

Honey

PROPERTIES/ACTIONS
- Helps insomnia
- Treats fungal infections
- Aids healing

PARTS USED
- Bees' honey

HONEY DRESSING
for wounds

honey
gauze bandage

Spread some honey onto a gauze bandage and apply it to the wound. The amount of honey used depends on the amount of fluid exuding from the wound. Large amounts of exudate require substantial amounts of honey. Reapply the dressing as necessary.

Ancient societies around the world used honey as an energy food. It has evolved as a unique and powerful remedy for a wide variety of complaints.

So prized was the food of bees that the Romans used it instead of gold to pay their taxes. Today, honey has become known as "liquid gold" with nutritive and healing properties.

Composed of 38 per cent fructose, 31 per cent glucose, 1 per cent sucrose and 9 per cent other sugars, honey is the only natural sweetener that requires no additional refining or processing. It helps with any tendency towards hypoglycaemia that may contribute towards insomnia and mood swings. It also provides many nutritional substances, including vitamin B6, thiamin, riboflavin, pantothenic acid, and trace amounts of minerals such as calcium, copper, iron, magnesium, manganese, phosphorus, potassium, sodium and zinc.

Honey is a recognized antioxidant and a powerful, broad-spectrum antibiotic with both anti-fungal and anti-microbial properties, acting against organisms that create the *Staphylococcus* virus and candida infections. Honey also contains an amazing substance called propolis, which is a natural antibacterial that helps to prevent and treat coughs and colds, as well as stomach disorders. The antibacterial content found in Manuka honey of New Zealand has been shown to kill the *Helicobacter pylori* bug that causes stomach ulcers, while unfiltered honey contains pollen grains and helps hayfever.

Used topically, honey has a powerful antiseptic effect for the treatment of ulcers, burns and wounds. It has an anti-inflammatory action, reducing swelling and pain, and by stimulating the regrowth of tissue under the skin's surface, honey helps the healing mechanism.

In ancient Greece the alcoholic honey drink mead was regarded as the drink of the gods.

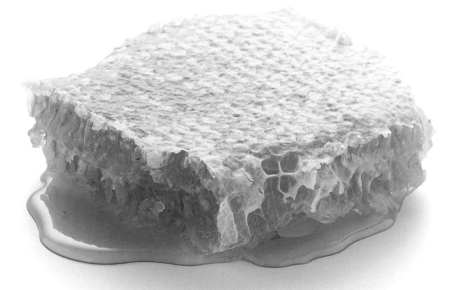

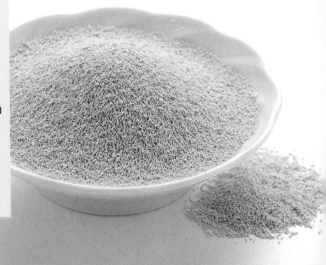

Brewer's Yeast

Containing almost 50 per cent protein, lecithin and unrivalled levels of B-complex vitamins, together with valuable minerals, brewer's yeast has long been used for its medicinal properties.

Brewer's yeast is a valuable remedy for fatigue and stress-related symptoms. It is rich in the nucleic acid RNA, as well as zinc, which are both vital to the immune system. Used topically in a compress, brewer's yeast is healing for skin complaints. Holding up to 70 per cent moisture, it is excellent for regenerating healthy tissue.

PROPERTIES/ACTIONS
- Treats fatigue
- Boosts immunity
- Heals the skin

PARTS USED
- Dried brewer's yeast

BREWER'S YEAST COMPRESS *for skin complaints*

225g (8oz/1 cup) powdered brewer's yeast
warm water
cotton cloth
small blanket

Combine the brewer's yeast with warm water to make a soft, moist paste (about the consistency of mustard). Spread onto the cotton cloth and apply to the affected area. Cover with the blanket and leave in place until the paste begins to dry. Remove, flush the area with cold water and allow to dry. Repeat according to symptoms.

Black Strap Molasses

Dark, sticky and rich in flavour, black strap molasses is an old-fashioned natural sweetener with high levels of nutrients.

Black strap molasses is rich in iron and is a fantastic remedy for rebuilding the blood and fighting against anaemia and fatigue. It also contains calcium, copper, manganese, potassium and magnesium, which help to prevent osteoporosis, promote a healthy nervous system and muscles, and boost immunity. According to Chinese medicine black strap molasses moistens the lungs and treats dry coughs.

PROPERTIES/ACTIONS
- Rich in nutrients
- Treats anaemia
- Helps prevent osteoporosis

PARTS USED
- Molasses from sugar cane

BLACK STRAP MOLASSES BARBECUE SAUCE

125g (4½oz/½ cup) black strap molasses
250ml (9fl oz/2 cups) tomato sauce
125ml (4fl oz/½ cup) balsamic vinegar
juice of 2 lemons
85g (3oz/½ cup) brown sugar
cayenne pepper, to taste

Combine the ingredients in a heat-proof bowl. Place over a saucepan of boiling water, stirring occasionally, until reduced by a third. Remove from the heat and allow the sauce to thicken as it cools.

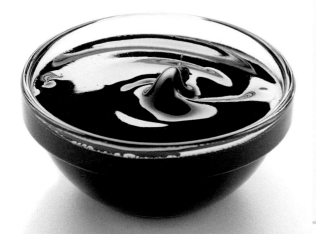

Rock Salt

PROPERTIES/ACTIONS
- Expectorant
- Treats respiratory troubles
- Good for sore throats
- Builds immunity
- Conditions the skin

PARTS USED
- Rock salt crystals

SALT-WATER NASAL WASH *for nasal symptoms*

250ml (9fl oz/1 cup) warm water
pinch of salt
pinch of ground turmeric (optional)

Mix together the ingredients and pour into a small jug with a narrow spout. Inhale the salty mixture (through the narrow spout) up one nostril. Tilt your head back and allow the mixture to drain into the back of your mouth before spitting it out, then do the same with the other nostril. Repeat up to 5 times a day with symptoms.

Since the beginning of Greek medicine, salt has commonly been used as an inhalant for respiratory diseases, and topically for the skin.

Salt has expectorant powers and may relieve coughs, colds and sinusitis. The inhalation of steam from salt water has anti-inflammatory effects, offering further relief from respiratory symptoms, and salt can be used as a sore-throat gargle. Salt baths increase circulation and the elimination of toxins. They may condition the skin, relieve eczema, treat tired muscles and build up resistance to disease.

The ancient Greeks first noted that eating salty food promoted basic body health.

Tofu

One of the most convenient vegetarian forms of protein, tofu works well in everything from smoothies to stir-fries.

Also known as bean curd, tofu is a versatile, low-fat food jam-packed with nutrients. Like all soya products, it is rich in phytoestrogens that help to regulate hormone levels, and calcium to build strong bones. Tofu is a good source of omega-3 fatty acids and fibre, which both help to stave off food cravings. It also contains an isoflavone called genistein, which seems to promote fat loss by reducing the size and number of fat cells.

Soft tofu blends easily in smoothies and desserts; firm tofu works well in main meals.

NUTRIENTS

Vitamins A, K; calcium, copper, iron, magnesium, manganese, phosphorus, potassium, selenium; omega-3 and -6 essential fatty acids

BLUEBERRY AND TOFU MOUSSE *serves 4*

200g (7oz) silken tofu
250g (9oz/1⅔ cups) blueberries
85g (3oz/¾ cup) ground almonds
1 tsp ground cinnamon
1 tsp lemon juice
2 tsp toasted, flaked almonds

Blend the tofu and blueberries in a food processor. Add the ground almonds, cinnamon and lemon juice. Spoon the mousse into four bowls and sprinkle over the almond flakes.

Miso

NUTRIENTS

Vitamins B1, B2, B3, B5, B6, K, beta-carotene, folic acid (folate); calcium, copper, iron, magnesium, manganese, phosphorus, potassium, selenium, sodium, zinc

Miso does more than just add flavour to soups and stews, it notches up their nutrient rankings, too.

A naturally fermented paste, miso is made from soya beans, sea salt and a yeast mould called *koji*. A handy store-cupboard staple, it is ideal for spicing up soups, sauces and stews. Miso is an excellent source of protein, and boasts a host of minerals, including manganese, which strengthens nerves, bones and muscles, and phosphorus, necessary for the metabolism of fats, protein and glucose.

MISO SANDWICH SPREAD *serves 1*

1 tbsp miso
1 tbsp tahini
1 garlic clove, crushed

Mix all the ingredients together well in a small bowl. Use over warm crusty wholemeal bread or use as a tasty substitute for butter in sandwiches.

Dark miso contains more protein and essential fatty acids than lighter varieties.

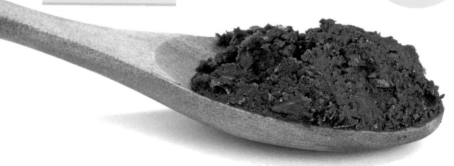

Coffee

PROPERTIES/ACTIONS
- Brain stimulant
- Treats asthma
- Diuretic
- Purgative

PARTS USED
- Beans

COFFEE POULTICE
for insect bites & bruises

**50g (1¾oz/⅓ cup) coffee
  grounds
gauze bandage**

Soak the coffee in 60ml (2fl oz/
¼ cup) water, then spread
directly onto the affected area.
Cover and wrap with the gauze
bandage. Leave for several
hours, or until the coffee dries.

Coffee first arrived in Europe from Arabia in the
1600s, when it was valued as a medicine, and has
since evolved as a popular beverage.

Containing caffeine, coffee is a proven pick-me-up that stimulates
the brain and improves mental performance and concentration. It
can also bolster mood and mild depression. With its ability to relax
the bronchial muscles, coffee is helpful to some asthmatics. It can
also offer relief from migraine.

Coffee is a diuretic and can therefore relieve constipation. It
may also help to prevent cancer. A poultice of wet coffee grounds
can speed the healing of insect bites and bruises.

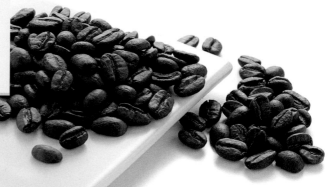

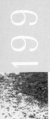

Green Tea

Not just a refreshingly different brew, green tea is packed with powerful healing nutrients.

NUTRIENTS
Vitamin C; flavonoids

GREEN TEA FACTS
• Although green tea contains less caffeine than black tea, it still has stimulant effects and should be avoided close to bedtime or by those prone to anxiety.

• The ancient Greeks called tea "the divine leaf", and used it to treat respiratory complaints, such as colds and asthma.

• Green tea's ability to fight free radicals means it has powerful anti-ageing properties.

Green tea comes from the same plant, *camellia sinensis*, as ordinary black tea, but has been processed differently, leaving important nutrients intact. It is grown in high areas in countries with warm, wet climates such as Japan and India, but China is the biggest tea producer. The medicinal properties of green tea have been recognised there for over 4,000 years. It has a fresh, astringent flavour.

GREEN TEA'S IMMUNITY-BOOSTING PROPERTIES
This humble hot drink is a powerhouse of polyphenols – potent antioxidant flavonoids which neutralise damaging free radicals, helping to prevent disease. Tea's polyphenols include catechins, which counteract cancer-causing agents. It is also anti-inflammatory

and can prevent flare-ups of allergic conditions such as asthma. Green tea can help to lower blood pressure and cholesterol and stop the hardening of the arteries, reducing the risk of heart disease and strokes. Its anti-bacterial abilities mean it can fight tooth decay and gum disease.

USING GREEN TEA

In order to maximise the benefits of green tea, you need to drink it strong – leave it to brew for at least five minutes. However, some people find this too bitter and compromise by drinking it weaker. Green tea is available both loose and in teabags, with natural flavourings such as lemon and apple, and herbs such as digestion-soothing peppermint and brain-boosting ginkgo biloba added for further health benefits. Choose high quality gunpowder green tea if possible, preferably organic. Green tea is best drunk without milk, but you could add lemon or honey to taste.

MOROCCAN MINT TEA
serves 4

2 tbsp gunpowder green tea
1 litre (35fl oz/4¼ cups) boiling
   water
good bunch of mint
brown sugar, to taste

Place the tea in a teapot, cover with boiling water and leave to steep for 3 minutes. Wash the mint, pull out a few sprigs to save for each serving, then add the rest to the pot and leave for a further 5 minutes. Pour into glasses, adding sugar if desired, and decorate with the saved sprigs of mint.

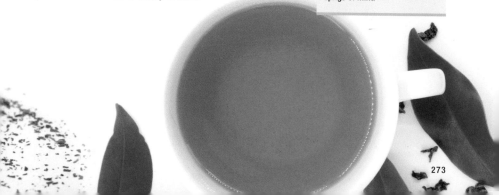

273

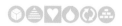

Wheatgrass

NUTRIENTS

Vitamin A, B-vitamins, vitamins C, E, K; calcium, magnesium, manganese, phosphorus, potassium, selenium, zinc; chlorophyll

Positively bursting with nutrients, wheatgrass is an elixir of youthfulness.

Wheatgrass contains all the vitamins except vitamin D. It's also rich in enzymes, minerals and proteins. This makes it good for everything from the nervous system to the circulatory system, to eye health and skin elasticity. Wheatgrass is said to help to prevent tooth decay, and to stop hair going grey. Its high chlorophyll content boosts production of blood. Wheatgrass also helps to combat the toxins in the body, which left unchecked, can accelerate the ageing process.

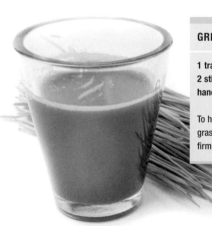

GREEN GARDEN COCKTAIL

1 tray fresh wheatgrass
2 sticks celery
handful of parsley

To harvest the wheatgrass, grasp a small bundle of blades firmly, and with a sharp knife, cut them off above the compost level. Rinse all the ingredients in cold water and feed them into a masticating juicer. Repeat with 2–3 more bundles of wheatgrass. Drink about 2 tbsp each day on an empty stomach.

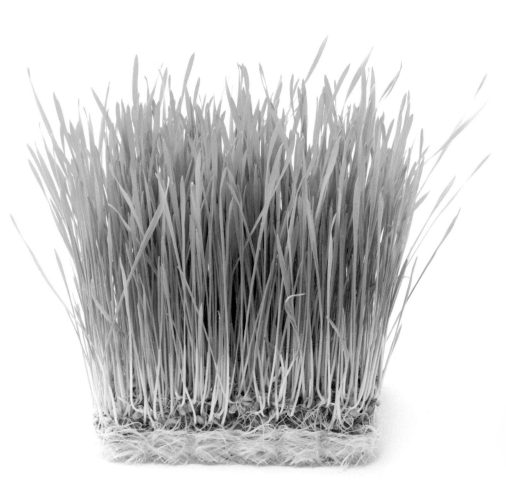

INDEX